The Family Guide to Children's Ailments

The Family Guide to Children's Ailments

Richard West MD, FRCP, DCH

Contributions by Michael Watkinson, MRCP

HAMLYN

London   New York   Sydney   Toronto

A Quarto book

Published by the Hamlyn Publishing Group Limited
London · New York · Sydney · Toronto
Astronaut House, Feltham, Middlesex, England

ISBN 0 600 384853
This book was designed and produced by
Quarto Publishing Limited, 32 Kingly Court, London W1

Typeset in Great Britain by QV Typesetting Limited
Printed in Hong Kong by Lee Fung Asco Limited
Origination by Hong Kong Graphic Arts Services Centre

Art Editor: Nick Clark
Editors: Emma Johnson-Gilbert, Lucinda Sebag-Montefiore
Designer: Joanna Swindell
Art Designer: Robert Morley
Editorial Director: Jeremy Harwood
Photographers: John Wyand, Ian Howes
Illustrators: Roger Twinn, Dave Worth, Simon Roulstone,
Edwina Keene, Dave Mallott, Paul Cooper
Charlotte Styles, David Lawrence, Chris Forsey, Hussien Hussien

To Jenny, Simon, Sarah and Sophie

Contents

Words and phrases which are italicized indicate a cross-reference.
Words and phrases in small capitals indicate an entry in the glossary on pages 150-165.

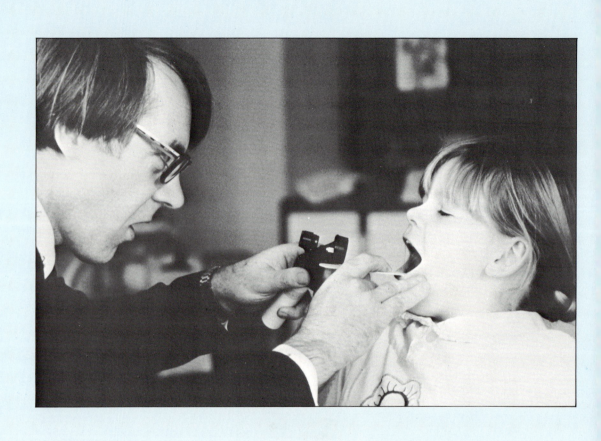

Foreword

A healthy child is not just one who
is free from illness. A child is growing and developing
in body, mind and personality all the time and full
health includes achieving optimum potential. Parents
play a major role in keeping children healthy by
providing for their physical needs, giving them plenty
of affection and emotional support and providing
them with stimulation and opportunities for learning.
This book aims to help parents in caring for their
children. Information is given on common childhood
illnesses, on maintaining the general well-being
of the child, on first aid and accident prevention
and on the organization of health care services. It will
therefore amplify and supplement information and
advice given by the doctor and other health care
workers who help to look after the child. For purely
practical reasons, the male pronoun has been used
throughout the text.

Richard West.

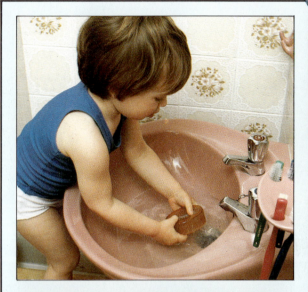

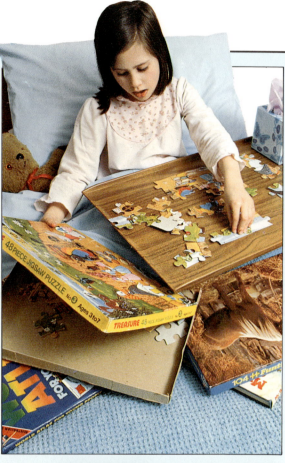

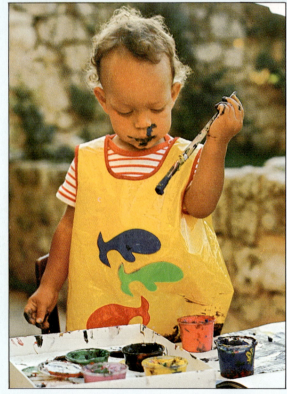

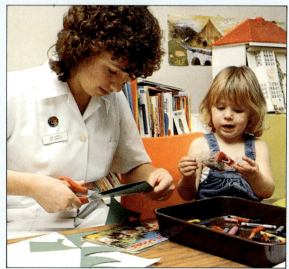

Section One:
Health and Your Child

Parents need to think about their child's health frequently and not only when the child is ill. This means considering all aspects of preventive medicine — accident prevention alone requires constant vigilance of the child.

Good health for children is cultivated by providing them with a loving home, which is both stimulating and supportive, and by giving them an appropriate and adequate diet. In addition parents should choose a doctor and arrange for regular health checks and immunization for their children.

Health care for children

THE MEDICAL CARE AVAILABLE for your child will be largely dependent upon where you live. Each country has a different system and the provisions under that system will probably vary between cities, smaller towns and country communities. Wherever you live, the key figure in your child's health will be a local doctor and preferably one to whom you can return over the years as your child develops. In addition you will probably make use of child health clinics, or well child clinics.

It is helpful if you have some understanding, both of the health needs of children, and of the services which are available to meet these needs. This section acts as a basic guide.

Choosing a doctor

There are a few important things to consider when selecting a family doctor. You need a doctor who is local and easy to get to see. Illness in childhood is often acute, and you want to be sure that your child does not have to wait a long time for an appointment and can be seen urgently if necessary.

There may be times when you need a home visit, if your child is too ill to be taken to the doctor; make sure your home is within the area your doctor will visit. But most important, you need a doctor with whom you feel you can talk freely and who has a special interest in children.

If you find you are not getting on well with your doctor, consider whether a change would be an improvement. The health and well-being of your child may depend on your doctor, so choose someone you like and have confidence in.

When to consult your doctor

Whenever you are worried about the health of your child, you should consult your doctor. An important part of a family doctor's job is to relieve family anxieties, so do not feel inhibited about contacting your doctor if you are worried. Even if the child does not seem ill, unexplained fever or persistent symptoms such as cough, noisy breathing or vomiting, may be reasons for seeking advice. Diarrhoea, particularly if accompanied by vomiting, may be serious in babies and young children as they can rapidly become deyhdrated and this demands a medical opinion.

Many doctors would rather see a sick child in their surgery or office, where all facilities are ready to hand, than make a home visit. If, however, you think your child could be infectious, or is too ill to be taken out, ask the doctor to call and see the child at home.

How doctors work

Children need a doctor when they are ill, or when parents are worried about their health. It is also

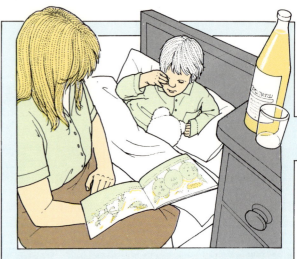

When a child becomes ill

Some childhood illnesses are trivial and do not need consultation with a doctor. Providing the child does not appear particularly unwell and is eating and drinking normally, mild infections, such as coughs and colds, can readily be managed at home.

Hospital admittance In hospital the child will be seen and examined by a specialist who will decide on the best treatment for the problem. The specialists a child may be referred to are as follows:

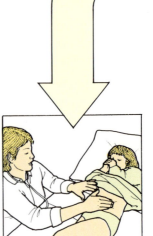

A paediatrician is a specialist in the medical care of children. As well as knowing about diseases, he has special knowledge of the health, growth and development of children.

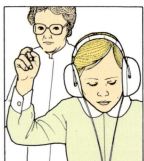

An audiologist is concerned with hearing and its problems. Special skills are needed to do detailed hearing tests on young children.

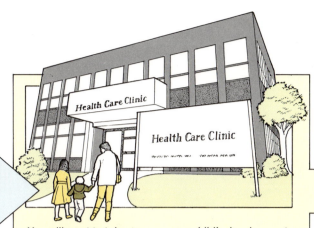

You will want to take your child to the doctor if he or she has become ill. You may also from time to time want medical advice on anything you have noticed which you may think is wrong or abnormal. If your child's development seems delayed or behaviour is difficult, the doctor should be consulted, and throughout childhood he should also attend a clinic for regular physical and developmental checks.

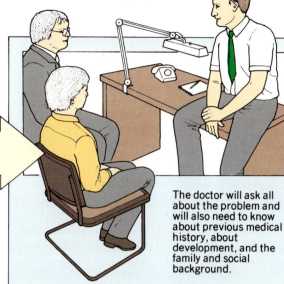

The doctor will ask all about the problem and will also need to know about previous medical history, about development, and the family and social background.

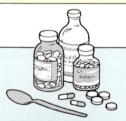

Prescriptions For most minor ailments, the doctor will prescribe medication which can be taken at home. If the medical problem requires further investigation, the child wil be sent to an out-patients department for Xrays, or will be admitted to hospital for examination.

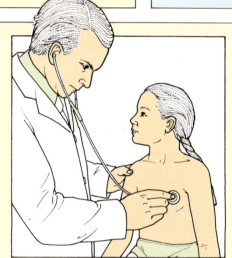

The doctor will then examine the child. Although this examination concentrates on the current problem, the doctor may take the opportunity for a medical check up at the same time. The doctor will probably make a diagnosis and recommend treatment, or suggest investigations. Sometimes a specialist opinion is required, or the child needs to be admitted to hospital for investigations and treatment.

The child will be weighed and measured. The doctor is likely to examine the heart and chest, feel the abdomen and look in the ears and throat. He may also look at other body systems.

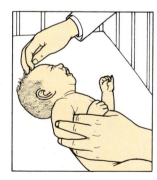

A dermatologist is a specialist in diseases of the skin and hair.

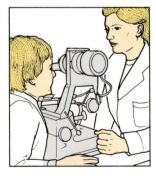

An ophthalmologist is concerned with eye defects and with squints.

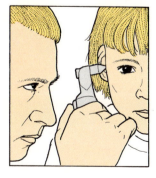

ENT surgeons (or otolaryngologists) see children with ear, nose and throat disorders. Children with recurrent ear infections, or sore throats may warrant specialist referral.

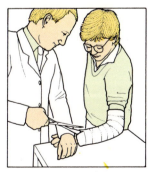

Orthopaedic surgeons are concerned with bones and joints. They deal with bone fractures and dislocations, and with deformities and diseases of bone.

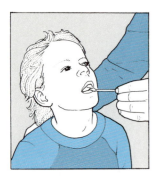

Swabs Swabs may be taken from the nose, throat, skin or other sites of suspected infection (see above). Sterile buds of cotton on sticks are rubbed over the area thought to be infected and these swabs are sent to the microbiology laboratory to see if there are any bacteria present.

Blood tests Blood can be taken from a vein or, if only a small amount is needed, from a finger or heel prick. It is then sent off to the laboratory for testing. There are a wide variety of different blood tests which look for abnormalities of either red and white blood cells, or measure the chemical constituents of the blood. A routine blood test, often called a Guthrie test, is done on all newborn babies to check that they do not have the rare diseases PHENYLKETONURIA or HYPOTHYRODISM.

Urine testing Analysis of urine to detect unusual constituents such as glucose, protein or blood, can be done readily in a clinic or at the surgery. Other tests, such as looking for urinary infection, require laboratory facilities.

Xrays Xrays which show the bones and internal organs are familiar to everyone.

Special Xrays using contrast media (dyes) to show up the internal organs are sometimes done on children. They are a barium meal to show the stomach and intestines, a barium enema to show the lower bowel, and intravenous pylography (IVP) to show the kidneys and urinary system.

important that they have regular, routine health checks for assessment of developmental progress, and for the early detection of any disabilities. These routine checks may be carried out by the doctor. More commonly they are provided by the local child health clinic.

When a doctor is consulted about an episode of illness, he first has to discover what is wrong. When he has made a diagnosis he can advise on management, including prescribing any necessary medication or other treatment.

The first stage in making a diagnosis is to compile a medical history of the patient. The doctor will want to know all about the symptoms and when they started. He will also be interested in details of the child's previous illnesses, immunizations, and the birth. If he does not know the family, he may well ask at the same time for some family and social background information.

Regular medical checks

Children should have regular medical checks by the family doctor, or the medical officer at the local child health clinic, and later by the school doctor. These are done at various ages, most commonly, at six to eight weeks, at six, twelve and eighteen months, at two and three years, and at school entry.

These routine medical checks provide an opportunity for the parent to discuss any health queries or anxieties with the doctor. The child is weighed and measured to make sure he is growing satisfactorily, and is examined for any conditions which may need a specialist opinion, such as a squint, heart murmurs, or *undescended testicles*. Coordination, vision and hearing are tested, and mental, emotional and social development is assessed. Usually the child will be developing normally, and the parents will be reassured. If, however, any problem is found, it can be dealt with at an early stage. The family doctor may arrange for a child to attend the hospital for an out-patient consultation, or to be admitted for investigation or treatment.

The doctor will then make an examination of the child, which includes such things as taking the pulse, looking in ears and eyes, examining the mouth and throat, listening to the chest, feeling the abdomen, and checking the nervous system. When the examination has been completed, the doctor may know what is wrong, or may have a short list of possible conditions which could be causing the patient's symptoms. Sometimes *special investigations* are needed to diagnose the illness, and sometimes the doctor will want to refer the child for a specialist opinion.

Prescribing for children

Once the doctor has made a diagnosis he will give advice on management. Often a word of explanation and

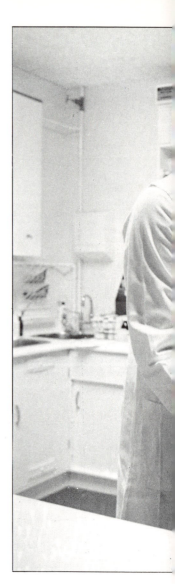

Health Centre In many areas community medical care is concentrated into a health centre. The centre will be staffed by doctors and nurses as well as by other health professionals and clerical staff. The health centre will arrange for regular developmental checks for children, and for all immunizations at the appropriate time.

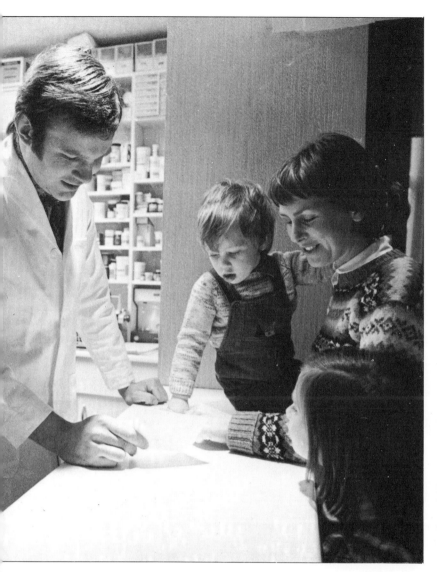

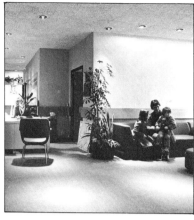

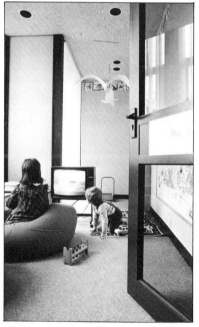

reassurance is all that is needed, and no specific treatment is required. For many complaints, the doctor will prescribe some medication.

There are an ever increasing number of modern drugs available to treat childhood conditions which formerly led to serious illness or disability in children. This medication has contributed much to the improvement of child health.

Young children have difficulty in swallowing tablets and capsules, so many medications are available in syrups or suspensions to make them easy for the child to take. These usually contain a lot of sugar. If the child is having medication for a long time, this can predispose to dental decay, so attention to tooth cleaning is very important. It may be worth considering an alternative way of administering the medication, such as using crushed tablets.

Powerful drugs have a greater potential for good than many older remedies, but they are also more likely to produce side-effects. The doctor has to consider the severity of the illness and any possible complications with his knowledge of the benefits, limitations, and possible side-effects of the available treatment. The use

and possible over-use of antibiotics is a frequent cause of parental anxiety.

Infection may be caused by either bacteria or a virus. Antibiotic treatment is of no benefit in viral diseases, but a wide variety of bacterial diseases can be treated with the many different antibiotics available. The virtual disappearance of some serious infections, including scarlet fever, lobar pneumonia, and of acute NEPHRITIS and rheumatic fever, has been largely due to the widespread use of antibiotics.

The most common harmful effects of antibiotic treatment are skin rashes, diarrhoea, and soreness of the mouth, but other side-effects are occasionally seen. The widespread use of antibiotics has led to some bacteria developing a resistance to common antibiotics. The use of antibiotics, therefore, is best restricted to patients with serious bacterial infections, to those liable to recurrent infection, and to small children and infants who are likely to have little resistance to infection.

Always remember to keep all medicines well out of reach of children, preferably in a locked cupboard, and when the child has recovered throw any unused medicine down the toilet.

Home nursing

A CHILD WHO IS ILL at home needs a lot of care, attention and reassurance. Consideration needs to be given to how best to provide that care and what should be done to aid full recovery.

Eating and drinking

Appetite is often reduced by illness, and unless the doctor has made a special suggestion for diet, parents are best guided by what the child fancies.

The child who has been vomiting or had diarrhoea will need fluid, and initially should be given watery drinks in frequent small amounts (see also page 50). Other children who are ill often take drinks more readily than solid food. Glucose or milk drinks are nutritious and help to provide energy for recovery.

As appetite recovers the child can be offered a choice of his favourite foods to help restore his strength.

Taking the temperature

The temperature of a normal child fluctuates during the day between 97-99°F/36-37°C, when taken in the mouth or rectally. A body temperature above this range constitutes fever, and in a child usually indicates the presence of an infection.

Treating a fever

When a child's temperature is very high, or is persistent you should consult your doctor to ascertain the cause

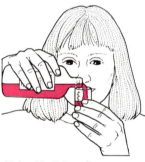

Giving Medicines For young children many medications are in liquid form and may be taken readily from a spoon or can be tipped into the child's mouth without protest. Medicines put in the front of the mouth can be spat out, so if the child is reluctant to take it, medicine may be given disguised in a small drink. Tablet medicines can be crushed between two spoons and the powder mixed with jam on a teaspoon, or blended with food.

Some useful things to keep in the family medicine chest (right) include a thermometer, a medicine spoon (5 ml), soluble aspirin or paracetamol elixir, calamine lotion for soothing sunburn and rashes, kaolin or other anti-diarrhoeal medicine, an anti-histamine cream for insect stings, antiseptic cream and solution for cuts and grazes.

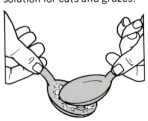

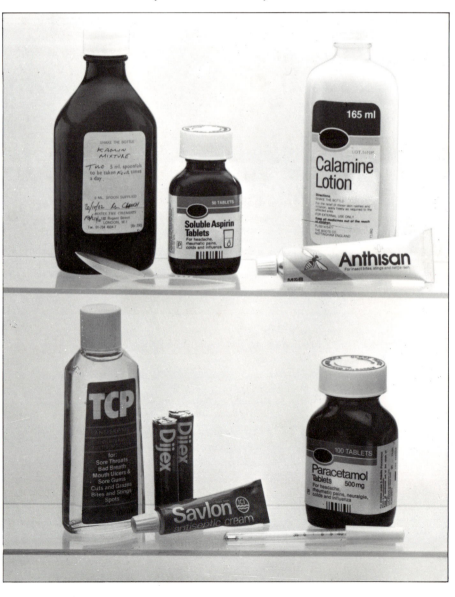

Resting in bed

When a child is feeling unwell he will probably want to stay in bed and is likely to sleep more than usual. If he has a cough or is short of breath he will usually be more comfortable propped up on pillows. Often a drink within reach is helpful.

As he recovers, the child will become more alert and active, and there is seldom any medical reason for keeping him in bed all the time. The child can be allowed up if he feels like it, and sitting in a chair is usually more comfortable than sitting up in bed. Both the room and the child should be kept warm.

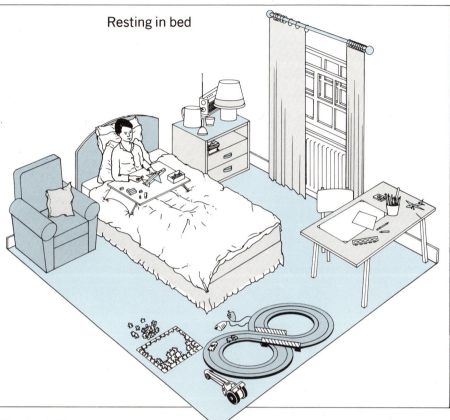

The clinical thermometer only registers temperature between 95-109°F/35-43°C. It has constriction in the bore at the bottom end of the scale to prevent the mercury column returning to the bulb before the temperature has been recorded.

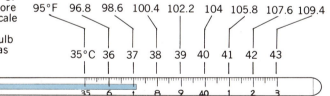

| 95°F | 96.8 | 98.6 | 100.4 | 102.2 | 104 | 105.8 | 107.6 | 109.4 |
| 35°C | 36 | 37 | 38 | 39 | 40 | 41 | 42 | 43 |

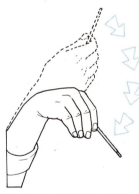

The thermometer must be shaken before use to get the mercury into the bulb. Keep the thermometer in place for at least one minute before taking it out and reading it.

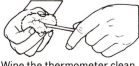

Wipe the thermometer clean after use. Do not put it into hot water.

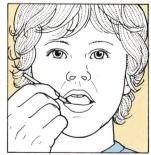

In the older child the temperature is usually taken in the mouth. Hot or cold drinks taken shortly before can lead to inaccuracies, so avoid giving them until after the temperature has been taken.

In younger children the temperature can be taken in the armpit (axilla). Axillary temperatures are usually about 1°F lower than mouth temperatures.

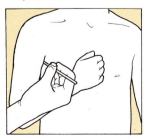

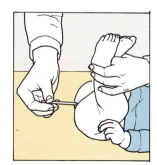

In babies the temperature is taken with the thermometer in the rectum. Take care not to hurt the baby by digging the thermometer in too far.

Keeping a sick child occupied

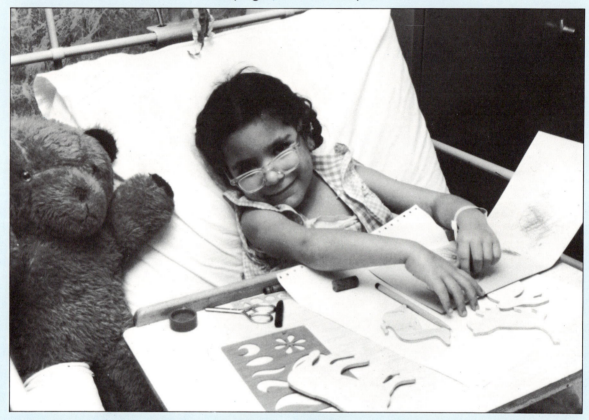

A child who is ill is less able to entertain himself than when he is well and is likely to tire easily. Sitting and talking to the child or reading stories, helps to make him feel secure. Television, radio and cassettes are all a great help and jigsaws, puzzles, dolls, construction toys and cars are suitable for the child to play with by himself. His attention span is likely to be short, and he will need frequent encouragement.

The following list of items and materials may prove useful and give you some ideas for keeping a child occupied when he is confined to the house because of illness.
It is a good idea to put a tray with legs, or a table, across the child's bed. This will make it easier for the child to eat, play games and do projects in bed.

Board games and **card games** can be played in bed, either by the child on his own or with friends and relatives. **Dominoes** are also fun.
Model kits can be made and painted. It is advisable to cover the bed with a plastic sheet and to give the child an overall if he is painting
Old magazines for cutting up and sticking down to make pictures and collages.
Pipe cleaners which can be

used to make amusing human and animal figures.
Paper and **pencils** for drawing.
Scrapbook and **glue** for sticking pictures, photographs, flowers, shapes or newspaper cuttings down.
Paints and **paintbrushes** (be sure to cover the table or part of the bed with a plastic cover).
Scissors
Empty boxes — e.g. cereal packets, egg boxes, cardboard tubes, kleenex cartons for making shapes and toys.
Video games and films can be obtained to amuse a child who is ill in bed.
Cotton wool
Felt and **kapock** for making soft toys
Wool and **knitting needles** for knitting
Books
Building bricks

It might be enjoyable for the child to **grow plants** by the bedside. They can be kept on the window sill, in a window box or on a shelf. Mustard and cress are particularly good because they come up so quickly, and parsley can also be grown quite easily.
Jigsaw puzzles
Coloured paper for cutting out shapes and making patterns
Shells for sticking down or making mobiles.
Soap bubbles
Needle and cotton, and coloured threads for needlework

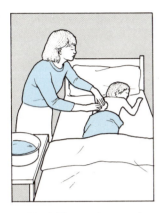

Bed bath First make sure that the bedroom is warm and that windows are closed. Remove the top bedclothes and help the child to take off pyjamas or nightdress. Place a towel underneath each part you are washing as you go along, to protect the bed.

As you wash, keep the child covered as much as possible and be sure to dry every area of the body thoroughly. You can also brush the child's teeth and hair. When the washing procedure is finished, help the child into clean nightclothes.

and to get appropriate treatment. Whatever the reason, being feverish makes the sufferer feel unwell, and in young children may provoke a convulsion (see page 116).

Lowering the temperature will make the child feel better. If he feels hot, most of his clothes should be taken off and he should be given plentiful amounts of fluid to encourage sweating. Paracetamol or soluble aspirin can be given to help lower the fever, and may be repeated six hourly.

If the temperature remains high in spite of these measures the child can be cooled by sponging the face and body with lukewarm water. This needs to be done repeatedly, but not for longer than half an hour, or more frequently than every two hours.

Giving medicines

There may be a problem in getting a child to take medicine that has been prescribed. For young children many medications are in liquid form and may be taken readily from a spoon or can be tipped into the child's mouth without protest. Medicines put in the front of the mouth can be spat out, so if the child is reluctant to take it, medicine may be given disguised in a small drink. It should not be put into a large volume in case the child will not drink it all. For babies liquid medicines can be instilled into the back of the mouth using a syringe. Tablet medicines can be crushed between two spoons and the powder mixed with jam on a teaspoon, or blended with food.

Nursing checklist

Keep the child comfortable — change the bedclothes regularly and make sure that the child is propped up and supported when eating or doing things in bed.

Give all medication, as prescribed.

Take the temperature if the child feels hot, and treat accordingly.

The child's appetite may be diminished if he is feeling ill, so try to encourage him to take nourishing drinks. Milk and glucose drinks are most beneficial.

The child will need plenty of care and attention. Keep an eye on his condition and stay with him during mealtimes if he appears to want company. Perhaps read to him if he is feeling drowsy.

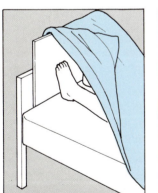
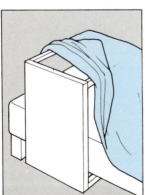
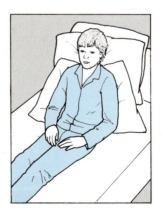

Comfort in bed is very important if you are ill and a child especially may be very restless. If a child is suffering from a back problem he may find it difficult to lie comfortably on a soft bed. The bed can be made rigid by putting a wooden board under the mattress. If there is injury to the legs or lower part of the body, the sheets

and blankets should be raised so that they do not touch the injured part. This can be done by wedging a piece of wood in a horizontal position at the end of the bed and putting the bedclothes over the top before tucking them in. Alternatively a table can be placed across the bed to raise the bedclothes out of the way.

Pillows should be arranged for maximum comfort when the child is sitting up in bed. Make a triangle with three or four pillows — this will give added support.

First Aid

For first aid treatment, safety in the home, prevention of accidents, bandaging and the first aid box, turn to pages 166-187.

Children in hospital

STAYING IN HOSPITAL CAN be a worrying time for a child. The surroundings are unfamiliar, many of the procedures performed are unpleasant, and may involve separation from family and friends.

If hospital admission is planned in advance, the parents have the opportunity of talking it over with the child and letting him know what to expect. Most children's wards welcome a visit before the admission so that the child can familiarize himself with the ward and meet some of the staff. If such a visit is not suggested by the staff of the children's ward, a phoned request will usually be all that is necessary to arrange such a visit.

For many children hospital admission is sudden and unplanned. This can be even more worrying for the child, and parents should be with him throughout the time he is being admitted until he is settled into the ward, so that they can reassure him by their presence.

The parents' role

Children may be anxious and upset about going into hospital, particularly if they are admitted as an emergency, without the parents having a chance to explain what is happening. They may also be bewildered at being cared for by strangers, and by the ward routines. With the right support from a parent, or other person close to them, many children can learn and become more mature as a result of the experience. They should be encouraged to talk about what is going on so that any fears can be recognized and dealt with.

Resident accommodation

For children under the age of five years, a stay in hospital can be very distressing, and this upset may persist for some time after they have returned home. If a parent or relative can stay in hospital with them, this does much to alleviate anxiety and distress. Most children's units have some accommodation for mothers but if resident accommodation is not available, you can ask if it is possible to stay with your child, as many wards can make provision for this, even if it is only a folding bed alongside your child's cot.

If parents cannot stay with their children, it helps for them to visit as much as possible. They should tell the child when they are leaving (even if it leads to a few tears), and when they are coming back, so that the child can take comfort in looking forward to their return.

Hospital routine

Children come into hospital for investigation and treatment of their illness, but they continue to have all the other needs of children as well — for feeding, washing, toiletting, playing, amusement, friendship, and affection. The nursing staff look after the child and all his needs while he is in hospital, and arrange for him to go to

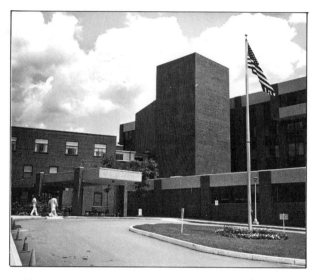

Children in hospital A hospital can be an unfamiliar and frightening place for children. If they need to be admitted they will want constant reassurance and support. There is usually a play area or play room for children in hospital where they can draw and paint, make things, play games and do projects. Nurses, play therapists and others will help in alleviating any anxieties, but having a parent or other relative resident with the child is a great help. If parents are not able to be resident they should make frequent visits. The picture (top right) shows a play area in hospital. It is worth remembering when preparing your child's things to take to hospital that they are often able to be out of bed and wearing their own clothes. The picture (bottom right) shows a resident mother nursing her baby.

any necessary departments for tests, such as Xrays. They also administer the medicine and carry out treatment ordered by the doctor.

On admission to hospital a nurse will show the way to the child's bed or cot, and explain the layout and workings of the ward. The resident doctors will take a history, examine the child, order any investigations necessary, and may start the child on some treatment. The doctor in charge will come back to see the child as often as necessary. He will certainly carry out a daily 'round' with the nursing staff to discuss each child and review progress. The resident doctor spends much of his time on the ward, and is readily available in an emergency.

The arrangement of the wards is obviously centred around the treatment needs of the children. They may also have play therapists and teachers who fulfil an important role, both in keeping the child occupied and helping him to express his feelings about being in

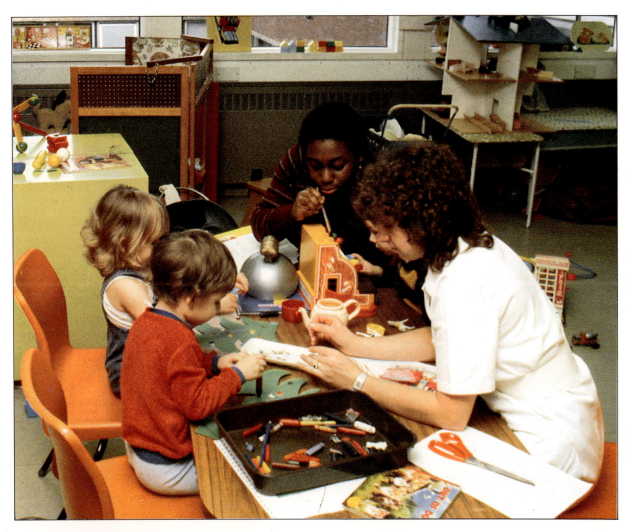

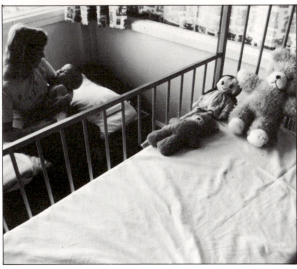

hospital. Nevertheless, there will be times when the child is bored and unhappy, so if a parent is unable to be resident with a young child, frequent visits are important. Most children's wards do not have any restrictions on visiting by parents.

Coming home again

Many children have some alteration in their behaviour on returning home from hospital. Fortunately this does not usually last for more than a week or two. Small children often become clinging and reluctant to let their parents out of their sight. They may be quiet and withdrawn, or quick to cry, and often the normal sleeping pattern is disturbed. Reversion to previous habits such as thumb-sucking or bed-wetting may occur. As the child regains confidence and a sense of security, behaviour gradually reverts to normal, and this is helped by understanding from the parents.

Who's who in hospital
Medical staff: The medical staff are organized into teams, sometimes known as firms. At its smallest a firm consists of a consultant who has overall medical responsibility for patients under his care, and a house officer (H.O) or senior house officer (S.H.O) who provides day-to-day care for the patients on the ward. Most firms also have a registrar, who has several years experience in his speciality, and who is probably in training to be a consultant. The registrar assists and supervises the house officer, but will also have other duties away from the ward.
Nursing staff: Each ward has a charge nurse or sister who is responsible for running the ward and organizing the working of the other nurses. Busy wards may have more than one sister. Staff nurses are fully trained nurses under the sister, and they will run the ward when the sister is off duty. Many of the other nurses will still be in training. There may also be some nursery nurses who have had a special training in caring for young children.
Other staff: A medical social worker will be attached to the ward. Hospital admission of a child may pose problems over finance or visiting, and the social worker can inform the family of the social services available to them.

A physiotherapist, may be involved with some children, particularly those with chest infections, asthma, and children with fractures and physical handicap.

There are also clerical, secretarial and domestic staff attached to the wards, each helping in making things run efficiently and smoothly.

Resident mothers Most children's units have some provision for resident mothers, although facilities may be limited. If your child is seriously ill of course you will want to stay, but children under the age of five, even if not very ill, may be upset by being in hospital and separated from what is familiar. Having his mother or another relative resident is of great comfort and support to the child.

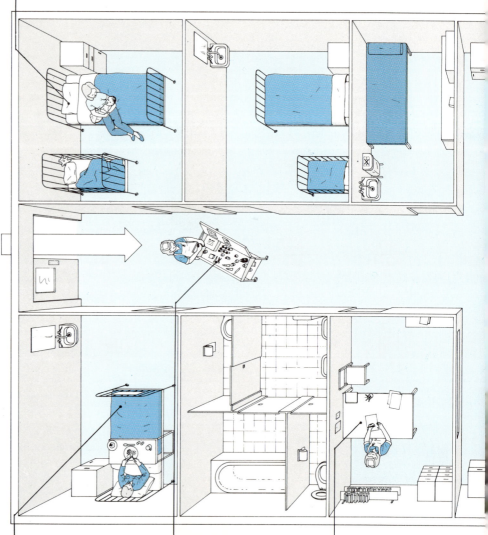

Quarantine If a child is put in quarantine it means either that his illness is infectious or that he is particularly susceptible to infection from outside carriers and so must be protected. Rules about quarantine will vary depending upon the nature of the infection. It does not necessarily mean that the child is refused all visitors, but all visiting instructions must be strictly followed.

Medicines The doctor will prescribe medication for many of the children in the ward. This may be liquid medicine, tablets or capsules. Sometimes medication needs to be given by another method such as inhalation or injection. The nursing staff do a 'drug round' at intervals during the day.

Sister's office The sister's office adjoins the main ward. There is usually a good view of the ward from the office. There is also a desk in the ward where nurses can sit and keep an eye on things if they are not otherwise occupied and at which the night nurse will usually sit.

Eating Children are encouraged to get up for their meals whenever possible and eat at the dining table. If a child has any food-related allergies or special feeding problems the nurse should be told so that the child's diet can be adjusted accordingly.

Visiting Frequent visits from relatives and friends, including brothers and sisters, helps the child to maintain contact with life outside the hospital. This is very important.

Curtains and screens around cots and beds can provide privacy for the patient. They are sometimes drawn when the doctor visits the child on a ward round and conducts an examination.

The daily routine in a children's ward is fairly flexible. A lot will depend on age, how ill the child is and whether special treatment is needed. The following timetable is a rough guide to the child's day in hospital.
06.00 - 07.00 Children wake up. A staff nurse checks the patients' condition and takes temperatures. Children who are well enough will get up.
07.45 Breakfast
08.30 Ward round made by the houseman or registrar.
09.00 Medication administered by nurses. Dressings, Xrays and physiotherapy for children who need them.

At some time during the day the consultant doctor may make a ward round. He will check each child's chart and general condition and talk to them about how they are feeling, and any on-going treatment.

12.00 Lunch
Children can usually make a selection from a menu. Special meals are prepared for children on special diets.
12.30 Mid-day observation by staff nurse or sister will probably be followed by a rest period.

Visiting hours are very flexible in a children's ward, unless the child is in quarantine. Friends and relatives are usually allowed to visit at any time.

18.00 - 19.00 Supper
19.00 Younger children will be washed and made ready for bed. Bedtime observation by staff nurse or sister. Older children are usually allowed to stay up later.

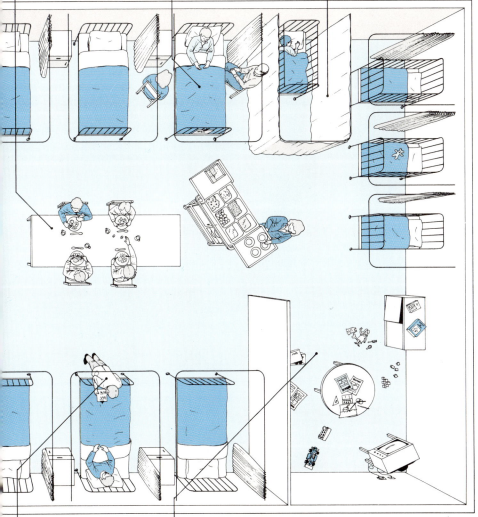

Ward rounds The resident doctors and the nurses will go round the ward regularly seeing all the children to assess their progress, decide on any necessary investigations, and plan the treatment. Nurses will also do regular rounds to take temperatures, to make beds, give out medicines and to make sure everything is going satisfactorily.

Play therapy Play is important to the child. It often allows him to express inner thoughts and emotions. Being in hospital can provoke feelings of insecurity and fear. An experienced play therapist can often recognize and help in allaying particular anxieties that have been identified when playing with the child. Playing doctors and nurses with a group of

children in hospital provides insight into their feelings.
Teaching There is a teacher attached to many wards. Children of school age can be given regular lessons and projects to occupy them providing they are not too ill. This helps them to keep up with school work if they have long or frequent spells in hospital, as well as providing a familiar structure for the day.

Things to take to hospital
- Towel
- Nightclothes
- Slippers
- Brush
- Comb
- Favourite toys and books
- Toothbrush
- Toothpaste
- Flannel or sponge
- Child's own clothes

21

Growth and development

CHILDHOOD IS THE TIME of growth. At the time of the birth there has already been rapid and remarkable growth from a microscopic single cell to a baby weighing perhaps 8 or 9lb. Throughout childhood the child continues to grow taller and heavier until growth finally ceases after puberty.

While this increase in size is occurring, there is simultaneous development of all other aspects of the individual including movement and coordination, visual skills, hearing and speech, and intellectual and social ability. All these will be considered briefly.

In the first year growth is usually assessed by weight alone. Babies tend to wriggle, so that measurement of length at this age is difficult, and often inaccurate. Doctors sometimes measure the size of the head with a tape measure to record another parameter of growth. As the child gets older measurement of height becomes easier, and both height and weight should be considered when the growth of a child is being studied.

Growth is most rapid in the first two years of life, and then it gradually slows down during childhood (see charts). At puberty there is another period of rapid growth which slows down as puberty ends, and stops completely when the final adult height is attained.

At birth, male babies tend to be slightly heavier than females (on average by about 1lb), and in early childhood boys continue to be, on average, slightly bigger than girls. Puberty is often earlier in girls than boys, so the puberty growth spurt occurs earlier and many may become taller than boys of the same age. Boys catch up and overtake in height again when they have their puberty growth spurt, and on average men are about 12 cm (4½ in) taller than women.

Normal children of any given age will show quite a wide variation in height and weight. Growth charts usually show a range of normality, which is more useful than just knowing the average height and weight for a particular age. Height may be determined by inheritance, tall parents tend to have tall children and short parents tend to have short offspring.

Growth is not only influenced by genetic factors, but is also affected by nutrition, by some of the hormones produced in the body, and by various diseases. Height in childhood is also influenced by the rate of maturation. Some children grow faster and appear taller than average, but enter puberty and stop growing sooner than usual. Others experience delayed growth and a late puberty, but do eventually attain a normal adult height.

Milestones in the first year

All dates are approximate
Controlling the head A newborn baby has no control over his head so it should be supported whenever the baby is handled, especially when he is being lifted from a lying position. By about six

Two months: The baby is beginning to be able to lift his head. The hand shows the grasp reflex.

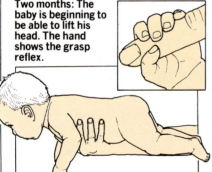

weeks of age he will probably be able to hold his head in line with his body for a short time. At eight weeks the neck muscles are getting stronger and when held horizontally the baby will be able to lift his head slightly. By about three months he can lift it quite high when held horizontally. By about four months he will be kicking his legs up and down.
Crawling The first step towards

crawling is when the baby can lift his chest by pushing down with his hands, and at the same time bend his knees up with a jerk. This occurs at about six months. Over the next couple of months he will move by rolling over and will support himself on his front with only one outstretched arm. By nine or ten months he may be pulling himself forward with his stomach on the ground, and by a year old the stomach will be off the floor and he will be mobile on all fours. It is important to remember that crawling is a stage that some babies do not go through since they become mobile on two legs first.
Sitting up With someone supporting his arms, the baby will sit from about four months of age and by about six months

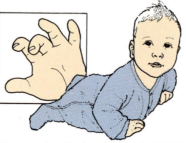

Four months: The head is now held high and the baby is kicking. The hands are open.

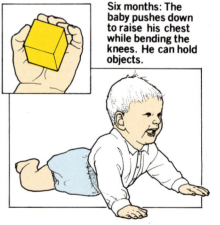

Six months: The baby pushes down to raise his chest while bending the knees. He can hold objects.

he can be propped up in a high chair. He will be supporting himself with his hands soon after this and by about eight months he will be able to sit up straight without support.
Using the hands Newborn babies have a strong grip, known as the grasp reflex, and usually keep their hands tightly closed. The grasp reflex becomes weaker over the first two months and by the third or fourth month has disappeared. At about this stage the baby will hold an object if it is actually placed in his hand, and will be able to put his hand in his mouth.

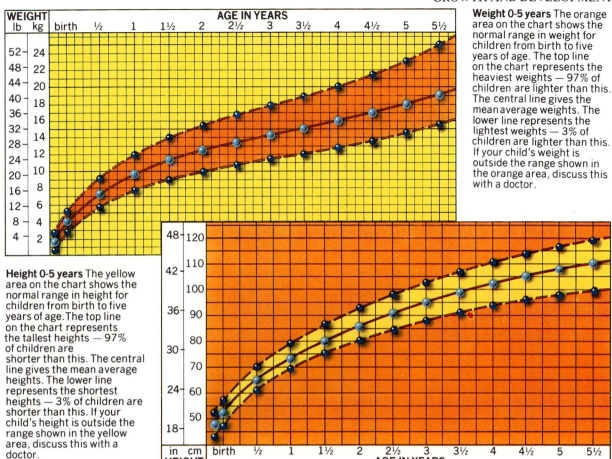

Weight 0-5 years The orange area on the chart shows the normal range in weight for children from birth to five years of age. The top line on the chart represents the heaviest weights — 97% of children are lighter than this. The central line gives the mean average weights. The lower line represents the lightest weights — 3% of children are lighter than this. If your child's weight is outside the range shown in the orange area, discuss this with a doctor.

Height 0-5 years The yellow area on the chart shows the normal range in height for children from birth to five years of age. The top line on the chart represents the tallest heights — 97% of children are shorter than this. The central line gives the mean average heights. The lower line represents the shortest heights — 3% of children are shorter than this. If your child's height is outside the range shown in the yellow area, discuss this with a doctor.

The baby is slowly learning how to coordinate his eyes and hands and he will gradually begin to reach out for objects which interest him.

Standing The big step towards standing up comes when a baby can take his own weight on his feet. This usually occurs in the ninth or tenth month, when he will stand while supporting himself with his hands. In the first few months, the baby will drop his feet to the ground when held and his legs will appear to be striding out. Then he

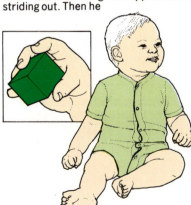

Eight months: Sitting up can now be achieved without support. The hands can pick up play bricks.

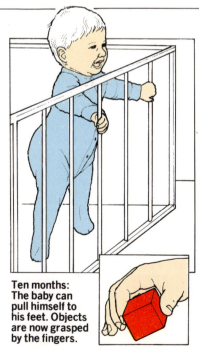

Ten months: The baby can pull himself to his feet. Objects are now grasped by the fingers.

will gradually take more and more of his own weight as the knees straighten. The ability to stand unsupported is closely linked to learning to walk.

Walking The first, tentative steps will almost definitely be taken holding an adult's hand for support. Following this the baby may proceed with a push-along cart or walking frame, until one day he begins to walk unsupported. At first he is bound to fall over easily and will move with arms outstretched and feet apart.

Children can begin walking at any time between about ten and eighteen months. They may take a few steps one day and then not try again for some time. Often if they are adept at crawling they will return to it even after learning to walk.

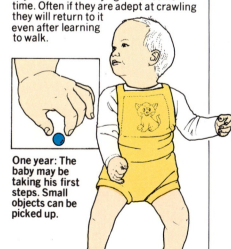

One year: The baby may be taking his first steps. Small objects can be picked up.

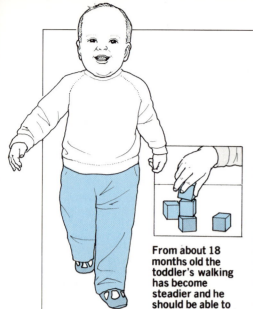

Milestones: One to five years

Motor Development Most children are walking well by about 15 months. Balance and coordination improve rapidly, and the child is soon able to walk quite long distances. During the second year the child learns to walk backwards, to run, and to walk up steps.

Jumping up and down is first done at about two to two and a half years, and standing still on one leg and hopping between the ages of three and four.

The child becomes interested in playing with a ball almost as soon as he can walk, and by the age of two will be able to kick and throw a ball forwards. Catching is more difficult and most children are not able to catch properly until the fifth year, even when something is thrown only a short distance.

By 16 months most children can put one building brick on top of another, and by two and a half years they are building towers of up to eight bricks, and enjoying knocking them down.

Between a year and 18 months children will start to scribble if given a pencil and paper, and by two and a half will probably be able to copy a drawing of a circle with adult encouragement. By four years first attempts at drawing people start. Although only the basic features, such as head and body are included in the first attempts. By the age of five many more features are included.

Language development At the end of the first year the child will probably use three or four words with meaning, but understand many more. From then on spoken vocabulary increases rapidly,

and between 18 months and two years elementary sentences are made by combining two words.

By the age of two the child will understand and carry out instructions, and be able to point to named parts of the body, or to objects in the room. From two years onwards the child's language becomes more fluent, with a gradual increase in vocabulary, and the

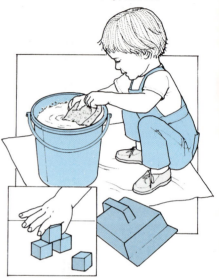

At about three years old the child will be able to build a higher tower and possibly construct a bridge with bricks. Many children of this age enjoy helping in the house with such chores as washing dishes, dusting and cleaning.

From about 18 months old the toddler's walking has become steadier and he should be able to walk unassisted. At this stage the child will be keen to explore for himself and may attempt to walk upstairs. He will also be able to bend down and pick things up and will enjoy building things such as towers of bricks.

The child acquires new abilities throughout childhood, with much of the basic foundations of motor, language and social development occurring in the first five years. The acquisition of motor skills is largely innate, but much of language and social development is learned and therefore influenced by the encouragement, support and stimulation given to the child by the parents and those about him.

Short children

If a child is thought to be small for his age, height and weight should be accurately measured. Using a growth chart it is possible to find out if the child is below normal growth limits. If a child is unusually small a reason should be sought.

Many short children have parents who are short. In such cases, the shortness is likely to be genetic and will not be helped by treatment. The family will be reassured that there is no underlying disease, but the child, particularly if it is a boy, may become very self-conscious about his stature and may be teased in school.

Short stature is sometimes caused by nutritional deficiency, but this is rare unless there is an intestinal disease leading to poor food absorption. Other chronic diseases leading to poor appetite may affect growth.

A deficiency of either thyroid hormone or growth hormone in the body will interfere with growth. If either condition is suspected, it can be diagnosed by a blood test, and if confirmed, treatment with hormone replacement therapy is possible.

Other conditions which may interfere with growth include severe congenital heart disease, renal failure, Down's Syndrome, ACHONDROPLASIA, emotional deprivation and many others, but usually the underlying disease will be readily apparent.

Tall children

It is very uncommon for tallness to be caused by disease. Usually it is due to a genetic predisposition to being tall, and requires no treatment. However, some girls are distressed at the thought that they will be excessively tall as an adult and seek advice. If predictions based on present height, skeletal maturity, and parental height confirm the likelihood that the girl will become very tall, it may be possible to reduce the final height by inducing early puberty with hormone treatment.

Motor development

Throughout childhood the child is developing new skills involving movement and muscle power. Some achievements, such as rolling over, sitting unsupported, standing alone, and walking are so distinctive that it is possible to say precisely when a child developed this particular skill. The tables (above and previous page) give some of the motor milestones of the first five years together with the age range at which they are achieved by most normal children.

It is important to realize, however, that each child is an individual and may have an individual pattern of development, so that the fact that one particular milestone is not reached in the average time is not necessarily significant. For example, most children go

The next stage, from three to four years, includes playing more complicated games and coordinating body and mind to do puzzles and to put on clothes and shoes without assistance.

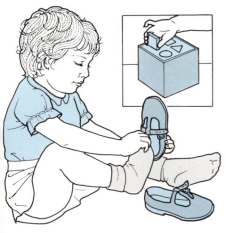

beginnings of use of adjectives and pronouns, plurals, and different tenses.

Opportunities for acquiring and using language are vitally important, and parents should talk as much as possible with their children.

Social Development Throughout the time that the child is making progress in motor and language skills, he will also be developing social skills. Between one and one and a half years the ability to use a spoon effectively for feeding is learned. At about the same

time he will also begin to acquire the ability to undress himself by removing a garment.

The ability to put clothes on is usually learnt in the third year, but requires quite a lot of supervision and help. Dressing without help happens in the fourth year, including the ability to do up buttons.

By 18 months the child will be imitating housework, and thereafter will enjoy helping parents in the home. Until about the age of three children may be worried by separation from their parents, even for short periods, but by three to three and a half are likely to separate easily to go and play with friends or attend a playgroup. From that time social interaction outside the family gradually increases.

Wax crayons and pencils can be used by most children from a year onwards for scribbling, but by the age of four or five the child will be using paints and producing pictures which are recognizable.

A picture drawn by a three year old (1) shows only the face of the parents. This is because the face is the first identifiable part of a human being that a child will see. By the age of seven the child will be drawing features and limbs, even if they are not yet quite in the right place (2). At about nine years old the child will have the proportions more in perspective and may have added details, such as a pattern on a dress or eyelashes to the eyes (3).

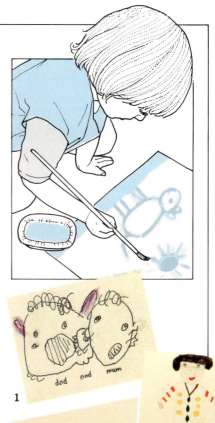

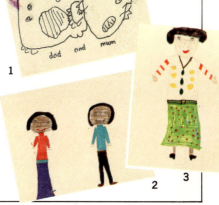

through a crawling stage, between sitting and pulling up to standing. A less common pattern of development, although just as normal, is to go from sitting to a stage of moving around in the sitting position — so called 'bottom shuffling'. Children who become bottom shufflers are often slower in standing and walking than children who develop through a crawling phase, but are in no way backward in their development; they are just manifesting an alternative normal developmental pattern.

Delayed development

If a child is consistently delayed in all locomotor achievements, it is possible that this is part of a more general delay, or there may be a problem with the strength or coordination of the muscles. Significant delay in achieving milestones is an indication that full development assessment should be made. This can be arranged through the family doctor or the child health clinic.

Visual skills

By about four weeks of age a baby can follow movement with his eyes, and will gradually show more interest in what is going on around him. Not until about three months do both eyes work together all the time, so

intermittent squinting is common in the first few weeks.

Once effective vision is established, it is a major stimulus for the child, and motivates action. Reaching out for objects, or crawling to explore something seen, encourages developmental progress. Control of fine movements, and learning to manipulate, depend a lot on the combination of motor movement and visual control which will result in steady balance.

Hearing and speech

At birth communication between mother and baby is established. This ability to respond to each other and meet the other's needs provides the baby with the foundation for the development of language later on. Inevitably part of this parent-infant interaction will involve the use of speech and the baby will gradually learn to take turns in making babbling noises and to identify and understand individual words. Gradually he will start to understand sentences and simple commands, will imitate sounds, and start to use words with a meaning.

Intellectual and social development

The development of the baby is very much influenced by surroundings. Of prime importance is learning to relate to a loving individual, initially the mother, and to form a

Boy's height This chart shows both the range of height for normal boys (between top and bottom lines) and the average height (middle lines) at different ages throughout childhood. There will be a period of rapid growth during puberty, so boys who enter puberty early grow faster than their peers at that particular stage. Those who experience a later onset of puberty will then catch up in height.

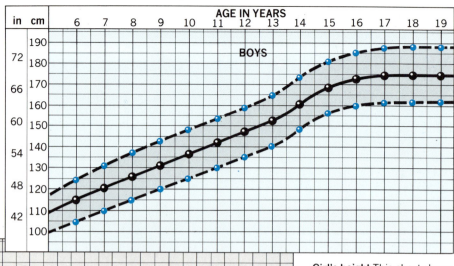

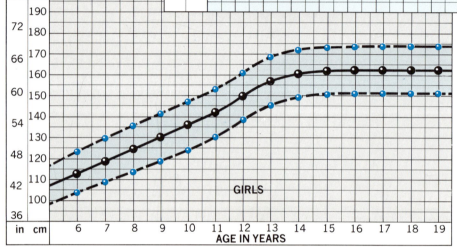

Girl's height This chart shows the range of height (between top and bottom) for normal girls at different ages throughout childhood. As children tend to grow according to the lines on the chart, for those under ten years old the chart can be used to predict the approximate adult height. Over the age of ten there is more variation in relative height because of differences in the time at which a child enters puberty. Prediction is therefore less accurate.

unique bond with her. When this bond is established, relationships will develop with the father and other members of the family, and later with outsiders. If the mother-child bond is constant, secure and loving, the child will have confidence and feel secure in making other relationships. As these relationships develop the child will be improving his ability to communicate, and will be building up his language. He will also be exploring and coming to know his environment. Learning and using his knowledge become part of everyday life and form the foundation of the development of intellect.

Parental role in early development
In all its aspects the development of the child is a dynamic process which is influenced by the relationships the child develops with other people, by learning about himself and his body, and by exploring and getting to know his surrounds. Whatever the child's innate potential for intellectual and emotional development, it can be enhanced by a caring and stimulating home environment, or depressed by insecurity and a denial of learning opportunities.

As well as being fun, talking and playing with children is one of the most valuable things that parents can do. Play provides many opportunities for communication and use of language; shared experiences, both new and familiar, broaden the child's horizons and help him to achieve his full potential.

Puberty
Puberty is the period of sexual maturation and, when it is completed, signifies the end of childhood. It starts as a result of hormonal changes in the body, and as the sex organs (gonads) grow and develop, they too release hormones into the circulation. These circulating hormones have widespread effects, altering the whole physical and emotional make up of the individual. At

Menstrual Periods
Periods do not usually start until the breasts and pubic hair are well developed and almost fully grown to adult proportions. Once puberty begins mothers should start to explain about menstruation. A girl will need to know why periods occur and to understand that she is entering the reproductive phase of her life. She will also need practical advice on sanitary towels or tampons, and on menstrual hygiene.

There are many useful booklets available which are written specially for teenagers explaining to them about puberty and sex. They should not be used as a substitute for talking together, but if a parent finds it difficult to discuss sex with the child these booklets will help by providing a starting point. Girls will receive some instruction at school and this can be discussed more fully at home.

the same time as these physical changes are occurring, the individual changes from a child largely dependent on his parents for security and support, to an independent adult.

Puberty in girls tends to start a year or two earlier than in boys. The first recognizable signs of puberty are a slight swelling of the breast tissue behind the nipple, and the growth of scanty pubic hair between the legs and under the arms. For most girls this stage usually occurs between 10 and 13 years. There is a gradual progression with enlargement and development of the breasts and increasing amounts of pubic hair. At the same time a slight growth spurt occurs causing weight gain and a gradual change in body shape. The first menstrual period usually occurs when the breasts and pubic hair are almost fully grown, probably between the ages of 12 and 14.

For boys, the first sign of puberty is enlargement of the testicles, followed by lengthening and broadening of the penis, increased wrinkling of the scrotum, and the growth of pubic hair. Hair starts to grow first around the base of the penis and this stage is usually reached between 11½ and 13½ years. As puberty advances a growth spurt occurs causing an increase in height and muscularity. By the time growth ceases, at around 15 to 18 years, the genitalia are of adult appearance, sexual maturity has been attained, and the voice has become deeper.

In both sexes, during puberty and adolescence, there is increasing interest and inquisitiveness in sexual matters, and a developing attraction between the sexes. Feelings are inevitably mixed, with both apprehension and excitement playing their part. It is a time of emotional turmoil, and this is compounded by the need to achieve independence from parents.

The adolescent lessens his dependence on his parents by becoming more assertive, and often argumentative. Family rows are common. Friendships, both male and female, are very important, and provide mutual support and encouragement in the quest for independence. When the adolescent is no longer dependent on the parents, either physically or emotionally, he has achieved adult status and often at this stage relationships within the home improve.

Precocious puberty

If signs of puberty are noted before the age of nine years in girls, or before the age of ten years in boys, puberty can be thought of as precocious. The earlier signs appear, the more likely there is to be an underlying hormonal or other medical problem. Precocious puberty is much more common in girls than in boys, and in most instances no cause is found; instead it seems to be an extreme variant of a normal process, and is referred to as 'constitutional precocious puberty.' As well as investigating to see whether there is an underlying cause for precocious puberty, doctors may sometimes give hormonal treatment to arrest the advance of puberty until a more appropriate age.

Delayed puberty

Children, or their parents, may feel that they are later than others in entering puberty. Even if this is the case puberty may still be within the normal time limit. However, if the onset of puberty appears to be excessively delayed, advice should be sought.

Usually delayed puberty is due to a general slow development, and both height and weight will be found to be less than normal for the age. If available, growth records may show that development has always been rather slow. In such cases, puberty is likely to occur normally, but later than average. In other cases puberty is delayed because there is failure of the sex organs (gonads) to produce the appropriate sex hormones. Such cases require full investigation and appropriate treatment.

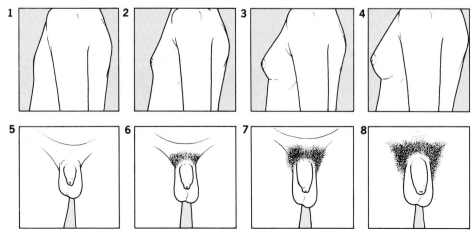

Changes of puberty The primary change at puberty is growth and maturation of the gonads, the ovaries in girls and the testicles in boys. At the same time there are secondary changes; in both sexes there is growth of hair in the pubic area and under the arms. In girls the breasts grow and gradually change shape, becoming fuller with maturity (pictures 1-4 left). There is also some broadening of the pelvis. In boys the scrotum and penis enlarge (pictures 5-8 left) and facial hair starts to grow.

Preventive medicine

CLEAN AIR, PURE DRINKING water, and good sanitation we now take for granted, but these factors together are of enormous importance in maintaining health. On a more individual level, there are several preventative measures which will help to keep children healthy.

Domestic hygiene

Gastro-intestinal infections are common in children, and are usually contracted through eating contaminated food. Storing food properly, hygienic preparation and discarding old food which might be going off, are all important. Teaching children to wash their hands thoroughly after toiletting and before meals is vital. Much of the time, hands which appear dirty will not carry any bacteria, but from time to time there will be contamination of the hands, and the only way to be safe is to insist on regular washing.

When a child is known to have an infectious disease he should be kept away from other children to try and prevent contagion. Some infections, such as chicken-pox, are highly infectious and all children will get them at some stage, but infection is more likely to be mild if only a brief exposure to the disease has occurred.

Immunization

A large part of the dramatic reduction in childhood mortality that has occurred in the last fifty years, has been due to the introduction of immunization against serious infectious diseases, such as polio, diphtheria, whooping cough and measles. Once a disease has been largely eradicated, the severity of it tends to be forgotten. It is only by continuing the immunization of children that many of these diseases can be kept at bay. The recent fall in the proportion of children immunized against whooping cough has led to a marked increase in the number of cases. Many of the children affected have had prolonged illness, and some have become desperately ill.

The benefits of all the commonly recommended immunizations are well evaluated, and the safety of the procedure is established. Parents should have their children immunized unless there are urgent medical contraindications.

See immunizations tables on pages 48 and 49.

Travel abroad

If you intend to travel with your child you should consult your doctor about whether any particular preventative measures are advisable. Your travel agent may also be able to advise you. No special precautions are necessary for Northern Europe, the United States, Australia or New Zealand. In other places, where sanitation may be defective, attention to personal hygiene is important and care should be taken in selecting food and drink. Immunization against typhoid is necessary for travellers to countries where typhoid is

A high standard of hygiene is essential in caring for babies and children to prevent the spread of infection. It is therefore important that food is stored properly, reheated thoroughly and discarded when it is going off. A baby needs to be kept scrupulously clean and feeding utensils must be sterilized before use (see page 141). As children get older it is vital that they are taught to wash their hands after using the toilet and before every meal.

Preventing yourself from harming your child

There will be times when you feel angry or frustrated with your baby or child, however much you love them. All parents experience such feelings. They may be provoked by the way the child is behaving, or by the demands of parenthood, or by other stresses affecting the family.

If a parent looses control because of the build-up of tensions at such times, the child may be harmed by being hit, slapped, shaken, or otherwise hurt.

A mother who is depressed may be helped by appropriate treatment from the doctor. If the baby is having feeding difficulties, or is crying a lot or not sleeping, the doctor or health visitor may be able to advise. When a child is demanding or difficult, a regular period in a day nursery may help both the child and the parents.

If you are worried that you may harm your child, or if you have already caused an injury, you should seek help. People often feel guilty about their feelings, thinking that others will consider them a cruel or unloving parent. As all parents at times have aggressive feelings towards their children, people used to helping families will understand your feelings, and will know how to be of assistance.

The person you approach for help may be someone in the family, or a close friend, but could also be the family doctor, a social worker, or the health visitor. It is much better to seek help in this way rather than risk harm to your child at some time in the future.

Dental care

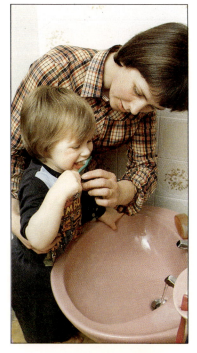

Tooth decay is common in children but it is largely preventable provided that precautionary steps are taken. It is important that not too much sugar is eaten, so it is a good idea to avoid giving too much right from the start so that the baby does not get a taste for sweet things. Snacks need not consist of chocolate, sweets and fizzy drinks; instead extra fruit and savoury things can be bought. Teeth should be brushed regularly and really well. Regular visits to the dentist are also important. It means that decay can be detected early and treated before it causes any trouble. The dentist can also demonstrate how to brush teeth properly and can tell you about fluoride tablets and drops which help to strengthen children's teeth against decay.

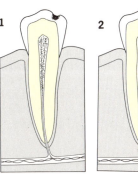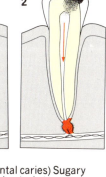

Tooth Decay (Dental caries) Sugary foods encourage bacteria to grow in the mouth. These bacteria form colonies, known as dental plaque, on the base of each tooth at the gum margins. The plaque bacteria gradually eat away the enamel (1). Once the enamel layer is breached the underlying dentine is attacked and rapidly eroded, giving rise to a cavity. If the cavity extends down to the pulp cavity, with its contained nerve, toothache will occur (2). Avoiding sugary foods, regular brushing of teeth, regular check-ups by the dentist, and fluoride all help in preventing decay.

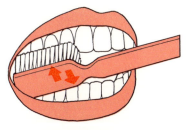

Every surface of every tooth should be thoroughly brushed. A vigorous up and down movement which produces a slight tingling sensation should be used to clean the front top and bottom teeth.

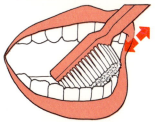

The back teeth and the chewing surface must also not be forgotten and must be carefully brushed. A toothbrush with a small head should be used.

in evidence. Cholera vaccine offers some protection against infection and is a compulsory requirement for many countries. However, it is not a substitute for careful personal hygiene. Anti-malarial prophylaxis is necessary in malarial areas, and the most suitable treatment varies with the part of the world to be visited. Infectious hepatitis is common in developing countries, and some protection is given for a few months by an injection of gammaglobulin.

Dental caries

Dental caries (tooth decay) can affect children badly. It is, however, largely preventable. Prevention is along three lines:
- Avoidance of dietary sugar
- Use of fluoride
- Regular brushing of teeth. Additional regular visits to the dentist are important to detect any caries early and to prevent it spreading.

Dietary sugar is ubiquitous in our society, so that even if sweets are severely restricted, the sugar consumption is still likely to be high. It is possible to choose snacks for children like crisps or fruit, rather than biscuits or cakes, to help reduce their sugar intake.

Fluoride can play a large part in preventing dental decay. Only in a few enlightened places in the United Kingdom is it added to the water supply, so most children have to be protected individually. The most effective form is for the child to have fluoride tablets, obtainable from most retail chemists, but they need to be taken regularly, from birth to about age 15. The dose is 0.5mg daily under the age of three years, and 1mg daily thereafter. In addition to taking fluoride tablets the teeth can also be protected by a fluoride coating applied by the dentist. This needs to be replaced every few months, but is an aid to prevention. Fluoride toothpaste is not as effective as fluoride tablets or the coating, but is slightly more protective than ordinary toothpaste.

See also page 71, At the dentist.

See also page 71, At the dentist.

Feeding your child

FOR THE FIRST FEW months milk is the only food necessary for babies. Breast feeding is the ideal method, and is possible for the majority of mothers. As well as nourishment, breast milk contains antibodies which help to protect the baby against infection. Bottle feeding is perfectly satisfactory using commercially available infant formulae, which have been made specially to cater for the nutritional requirements of infants.

Weaning, the introduction of solids into the diet, should not be started before three months, and there is no nutritional reason for introducing solids before five months, providing the supply of milk is adequate. Weaning can be started with baby cereal, fruit purée, finely minced or ground meat, and egg. Over the next few months the baby's diet will gradually become varied to include most of the things enjoyed by the parents.

Once past the toddler stage children will be on a mixed diet. Parents may well become confused about what constitutes a balanced diet in view of the differing dietary advice and warnings they are given, both for themselves and their children. Nevertheless, eating habits acquired in childhood often persist in later life, so establishing good dietary patterns may have prolonged benefits.

Types of food

Food consists of a mixture of proteins, fats, and carbohydrates, together with some indigestible matter known as dietary fibre. Proteins are essential for growth and repair of body tissues, but in an affluent society people eat far more protein than is necessary for body building. The excess is converted by the body to carbohydrates and used for energy.

Carbohydrates and fats are foods used by the body to produce energy for movement and for all the body processes. The body readily converts excess carbohydrates to fat for storage, or converts fat to carbohydrate whenever it is required. There are two main types of

Special diets

Special diets are sometimes prescribed as a treatment for a specific illness, or to help a child lose some weight. Listed below are some of the more common ones. Children should not be started on special diets without the advice of a doctor or dietitian.

Gluten-free diet
Children suffering from coeliac disease can not digest foods which contain gluten, a protein found in many cereals, especially wheat and rye. Foods containing gluten must therefore be excluded from the child's diet. Biscuits, bread, cakes, wheat flakes, ice cream, sausages, macaroni and spaghetti should not be eaten. Corn flakes, cornflower, rice, sago, tapioca and cakes and biscuits made with gluten-free flour can be eaten.

Low calorie diet
Obesity is a common problem in western society. Fat children get teased a lot, and may go on to become fat adults so it is important to take action if one's child is over-weight. Food, high in calories and rich in carbohydrates, such as bread, cake, candy, cereals, chocolate, honey, jam, marmalade, sugar, sweets, syrup and toffee should either be cut down or eliminated from a child's diet. Emphasis should be placed on protein foods — meat, fish, cheese and eggs — and fresh fruit and vegetables.

Diabetic diet
Children with diabetes have to regulate the amount of carbohydrates they eat. Small portions of carbohyrdates should be eaten at regular intervals so that no violent changes in the glucose content of the blood can occur. The control of blood glucose is likely to be better if most of the carbohydrate portions in the diet are eaten in the form of starchy foods (bread, potatoes, rice, beans) as opposed to sugary foods (sweets, chocolate, biscuits). Emphasis in the diet should be placed on high fibre foods such as wholemeal bread, salads and fresh fruit.

Exclusion diet for allergies
Some children are allergic to particular foods and these may provoke a reaction such as vomiting, diarrhoea, skin rash or wheezing due to bronchospasm if they are included in a child's diet. Sometimes a doctor will advise cutting out certain foods to see if any improvement occurs. Caution is always needed in excluding too many foods because a diet could be made nutritionally inadequate leading to vitamin deficiencies and other nutritional problems. It is therefore important that dietary exclusion is done under the supervision of a doctor or dietitian.

Minerals
Minerals are to be found in most natural unrefined foods — fruits, meats, vegetables, eggs, milk — and a well-balanced diet will generally provide a sufficient intake. Two minerals sometimes deficient in a person's diet are calcium and iron.

Calcium is essential for building teeth and bones and growing children need plenty of it. Milk and cheese are the richest sources.

Iron deficiency leads to anaemia and in a mild form this is fairly common. Iron can be found in meats and green vegetables — liver has a particularly high content. Preterm babies need to be given extra iron as they do not possess the required amount in their bodies at birth.

dietary carbohydrate — starch and sugar. Dietary fibre (or roughage), although not absorbed as food by the body, does play an extremely important part in the working of the intestines. A high fibre intake assists in regular defaecation, while a low fibre diet tends to be constipating.

In addition to these major dietary constituents of protein, carbohydrate, fat and fibre, vitamins and minerals are also necessary in the diet.

How much should children eat?
Both the quantity and type of food eaten may be important for health. If too little food is eaten, growth will be restricted and children will have little energy. Although common in the developing world, this is seldom seen in an industrialized society.

There is a wide variation in the amount of food that children eat, and in the amount that individual children need. Many children cause worry to their parents

because they have small appetites. Provided that such children are growing normally they are getting sufficient nourishment; cessation of growth is one of the body's reactions to an inadequate food intake.

Not all fat children eat excessively, but children who do overeat may become plump. If a child is inclined to be overweight, some regulation of the size of meals, and reduction in snacks between meals, may help to prevent the development of obesity.

The timing of meals is largely determined by family habits, but all children should start the day with some breakfast to provide them with energy during the morning.

What is a balanced diet?
Differing advice and warnings are given about the correct diet for both adults and children. It is important that a diet contains all types of food. Given a normal, varied diet, it is unlikely that any dietary deficiency will

Vitamins
Vitamins are special nutrients found in food and are necessary in small amounts for health. Vitamin deficiency is uncommon in the Western world because the majority of ordinary mixed diets provide a sufficient quantity. However marginal disorders are possible and growing children should be given a nourishing diet which provides them with an adequate vitamin intake; vitamin supplements are also recommended for infants. Besides a poor diet, metabolic disorders and other illnesses can lead to vitamin deficiency. Preterm and bottle-fed babies are also at risk.

Vitamin	Main Sources	Function	Comments
A	Dairy produce, e.g. milk, cheese, eggs etc, offal, vegetable oils, vegetables, dried apricots	Essential for good vision, particularly seeing in poor light	Children with cystic fibrosis and coeliac disease may be susceptible to deficiency.
B Complex	Dairy produce, meat, yeast, potatoes, cereal, wholemeal flour	Maintaining general health	
C	Citrus fruits, green vegetables, potatoes, rosehip syrup	Maintains condition of blood vessels and skin	Babies fed exclusively on cow's milk without added vitamins are at risk. The vitamin is destroyed by elaborate cooking.
D	Dairy produce, offal, fish liver oils, sunlight	Required to help body absorb calcium, strengthens bones and teeth	Deficiency can cause rickets. More common in vegetarians, and those on Asian diets. Children with cystic fibrosis and coeliac disease may be susceptible to deficiency.
K	Green leafy vegetables, vegetable oils, liver. Can be synthesised by bacteria in intestine	Essential for proper blood clotting	Newborn babies and children with jaundice are sometimes deficient.

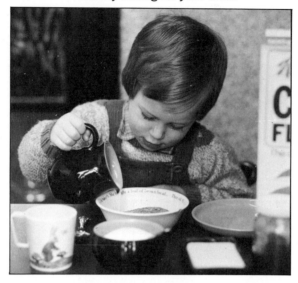
occur. There is no advantage in giving children extra protein since a normal diet will contain an excess of protein. A varied diet usually contains enough vitamins, but two groups of children are potentially liable to vitamin deficiency. These are babies in the first two years of life, who are growing rapidly, and Asian children who eat a traditional diet. All children should eat plenty of fruit and vegetables to ensure that they are getting adequate fibre in their diet.

In infancy growth is rapid, and children need relatively large amounts of many of the vitamins. Artificial baby milks are fortified with vitamins, but breast fed babies and infants on mixed feeding should be given vitamin supplements until the age of two years. Suitable multi-vitamin preparations are obtainable from child health clinics.

Asian diets may be rather low in vitamin D. When requirements for the vitamin are high, in infancy, during puberty, and in pregnancy, deficiency can occur. Milk, butter, margarine and meat are good dietary sources of the vitamin, but for some children vitamin

supplements are advisable up to the age of five years, and during the puberty growth spurt.

Sugar in the diet is a cause of dental caries (tooth decay). Sweets and candy are almost pure sugar, so are particularly damaging to teeth. Biscuits, cakes, and soft drinks also contain large amounts of sugar, and the amount consumed should be restricted. Starchy foods are a good source of energy and do not harm the teeth.

In affluent countries a great deal of fat is eaten in the diet. Ordinary dietary fat (so called saturated fat) tends to raise the level of cholesterol in the blood, and studies with adults have shown that some people with high blood cholesterols are likely to develop heart disease. In adults it therefore seems prudent to make a modest reduction in the amount of ordinary diet fat. The polyunsaturated fats (such as corn, sunflower, safflower oils and their products) tend to lower blood cholesterol. It is unlikely that the amount of dietary fat eaten in childhood has any effect on the incidence of heart disease in later life, but if healthy eating habits are established early they often persist into adulthood.

Exercise

WALKING AND RUNNING are everyday activities for children when small and, as ability and coordination come from repeated practice, such activity is necessary for normal development. As they get older, some children are on the go nearly all the time, while others are sedentary for long periods.

Parents should encourage an active lifestyle and, as the child gets older, participation in some sporting activity. Exercise improves a child's physical fitness, as well as developing coordination. Team games develop social skills as well as physical skills, and provide a structured introduction to competitiveness. Do, however, make sure the activity is safe, and the child does not become overtaxed.

There is a great deal of evidence to support the theory that a moderately active lifestyle promotes health and longevity in adults. The foundations for an active way of life need to be laid in childhood. In an age when many children are taken to school by car, and spend long periods watching television, it is important to encourage activities such as walking, cycling and swimming, as well as organized games and sports.

Developing skills through play

Young children get much of their exercise through play. As well as being an enjoyable and sociable pastime for children, playing games helps the child to develop control of his body, to gain physical competence and to heighten the use of sight, sound, touch and language. Play will also help the child to communicate and get on with other people and provides an outlet for emotion.

Balance and control

Movement	What is needed
Running	Space to run in, on different kinds of surfaces, indoors and outdoors.
Jumping/hopping	A few easy obstacles that the child can jump on and off, and over the top of. A skipping rope is a good idea for an older child. Games such as hopscotch can be fun.
Turning	Obstacles to run around, things to swing on and poles to turn around on.
Balancing	Lines to walk along, wide raised planks to walk and balance on.
Manipulation	Bending, stretching and twisting the whole body. Getting through and into small spaces and filling large spaces.

Movement in groups

Movement	What is needed
Games	Running and catching, skipping, stop-and-start games which require the players to move about and then become still, singing and clapping games in circles and lines, dancing games.

Controlling objects

Movement	What is Needed
Throwing/kicking	Soft balls of all sizes — small for throwing, large for kicking. Young children will not be able to aim very well, but can practise throwing for distance.
Catching/stopping	Beanbags, soft balls — large and small. Small balls can be caught in the hands or on the floor, if they are rolled. Large balls are stopped by the body.
Pushing, pulling and carrying	Boxes, balls, toys which can also be lifted up and down. Pushing and pulling games which can be invented and played by your children, or with them.

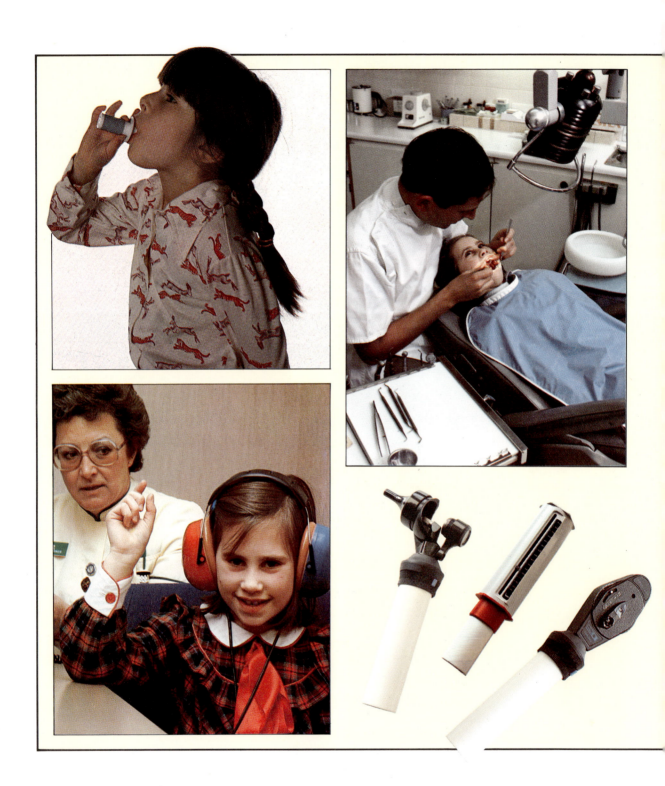

Section Two:
Ailments

The intention of this book is
to help parents to understand
the cause of children's ailments
and the investigation and
treatment of them.
It should not be used as a
substitute for obtaining medical
advice, but as information to
supplement that advice.
Section two covers both
common illnesses of children and
the more important
serious diseases of childhood
and adolescence. Other conditions
are described briefly
in the glossary on pages 150-165.

The newborn period

UNTIL BIRTH, THE BABY is entirely dependent on the mother for life. The foetus develops in the womb, obtaining oxygen and all necessary nutrients from the mother's circulation by way of the placenta. The circulation of the foetus carries the oxygen and nutrients around the body enabling the tissues to function and grow. Foetal wastes are returned through the placenta to the maternal circulation for subsequent excretion by the mother.

At birth the placenta separates from the womb, breaking the link between maternal and infant circulation, and the baby achieves independent existence. The newborn child suddenly finds itself in a strange environment to which its organs must adapt. Certain functions have to be established immediately.

The child must be provided with oxygen and warmth if it is to survive. Two processes are needed to supply oxygen: breathing to get oxygen into the lungs, and circulation of blood to distribute the oxygen to the rest of the body.

The digestive system must start working soon after birth so that the baby can feed, and the kidneys and bowels must function efficiently to excrete bodily wastes. Sometimes there is a delay or failure of the adaptations needed to achieve independent existence.

The first breath

At birth the baby enters a world which is brighter, noisier and colder than the womb. These marked changes set up nerve signals which stimulate the respiratory centre in the brain. The brain responds by initiating the first gasp, and the first cry. The first gasp draws air into the lungs, rather like a balloon being inflated, and thereafter regular respiration is established.

Usually a baby takes in his first breath within the first 30 seconds after birth, but in some babies the onset of respiration is delayed because of depression of the respiratory centre. The respiratory centre may be unresponsive because of sedative drugs given to the mother before labour, poor oxygen supply to the foetus, or for other reasons. If the onset of breathing is delayed the respiratory centre becomes even more depressed and there is then cause for concern.

The baby can, however, survive for several minutes without breathing. If the stimulus of birth has not started respiration, clearing mucus from the nose and

At birth the mouth and nose are full of secretions, and these have to be sucked out to prevent them being drawn into the lungs. This suction also serves as a stimulus to start breathing. Most babies start to breathe within half a minute of birth, and their colour then changes from blue to pink as the oxygen reaches the tissues.

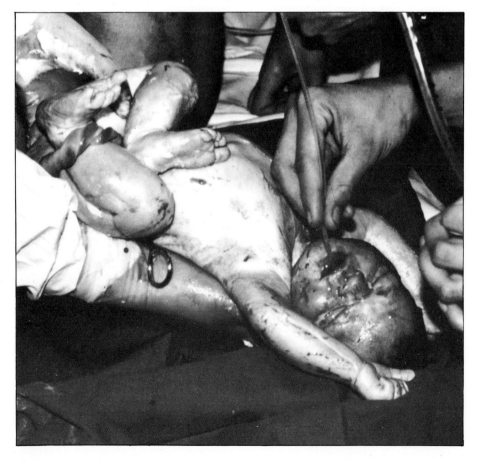

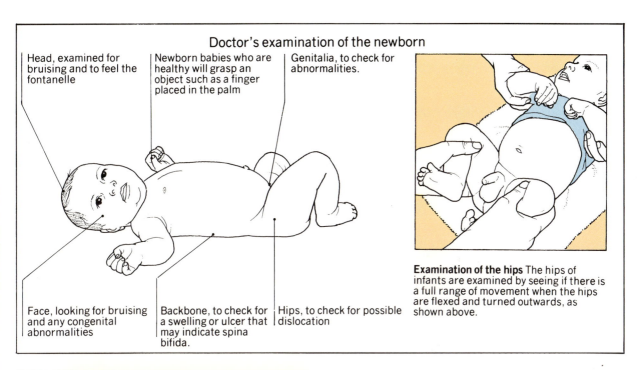

Doctor's examination of the newborn

Head, examined for bruising and to feel the fontanelle

Newborn babies who are healthy will grasp an object such as a finger placed in the palm

Genitalia, to check for abnormalities.

Face, looking for bruising and any congenital abnormalities

Backbone, to check for a swelling or ulcer that may indicate spina bifida.

Hips, to check for possible dislocation

Examination of the hips The hips of infants are examined by seeing if there is a full range of movement when the hips are flexed and turned outwards, as shown above.

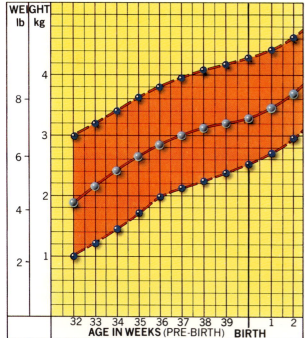

This chart shows growth in weight in the weeks before birth. Most babies will be within the outer lines shown. If a baby is below the bottom line at birth the term small-for-gestational age is used.

mouth using a suction tube may provoke the first gasp. If not the baby is moved to a resuscitation trolley which contains equipment and medication for immediate use. Oxygen is administered to the mouth of the baby so that if he does make a feeble gasp some oxygen will enter the lungs. If the delay in breathing is thought to be related to sedative drugs a stimulant injection may be given.

If these measures are not rapidly effective, artificial ventilation is started. Mouth-to-mouth ventilation can be given, but passing a tube into the windpipe (trachea) to administer oxygen is more efficient if a doctor skilled in the technique is available. In most cases natural breathing is established in a few minutes and the emergency is over. A small number of babies do not respond to resuscitation; they are said to be stillborn.

A stillbirth occurs either because a child dies in the womb before birth, or because breathing is never established after birth. The cause may be severe developmental abnormality or intrauterine infection, maternal illness, poor placental nutrition or oxygen supply, or premature separation of the placenta. Sometimes no cause is found.

For a couple to have a stillborn baby is a tragedy. Their loss brings to an abrupt end the months of waiting and planning for the new baby. Their grief may be accompanied by bewilderment. Doctors, and relatives have an important role in supporting the couple, and in helping them to come to terms with their loss. Many parents will also draw comfort from meeting other couples who have experienced a similar loss.

Care of low birth weight babies

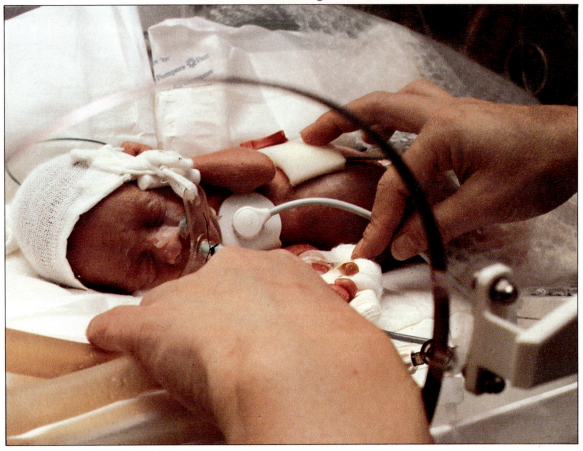

In preterm babies many necessary body functions have not fully developed. The earlier they are born the more severe these problems are likely to be. Low birth weight babies are likely to have some difficulty maintaining the correct body temperature and have problems with sucking and swallowing. Other common problems include breathing difficulties, jaundice and low resistance to infections. Small-for-dates babies are also likely to have low blood sugar levels.

Low birth weight babies are usually placed in a special care baby unit and cared for by specially trained doctors and nurses.

After the first few days (the period when problems are most likely to occur), growth and development of preterm babies is usually rapid, although not quite as fast as it would have been had they continued to grow normally in the womb until full term. Growth and development should be judged from the expected date of birth, not from the actual date of birth. So a child born four weeks early will be four weeks behind during the early stages of development. Most low birth weight babies catch up to normal weight very quickly and continue to make normal developmental progress. Babies born very small will usually have caught up by the age of two.

Neonatal Resuscitation Unit The mobile system (shown above) is on hand in the delivery suite to provide essential facilities for babies born with breathing difficulties. The unit contains oxygen cylinders for immediate resuscitation, equipment for ventilation and all the necessary medical instruments. The overhead unit is a radiant heater for keeping the baby warm.

Incubator Most low birth weight babies will need to be placed in an incubator to maintain their body temperature. Milk feeds may have to be given through a tube passed down the throat into the stomach. Sometimes drip feeding is necessary. It is routine in many units to continuously measure heart rate and respiration in small newborns. Unobtrusive monitoring machines record these vital signs and give a warning signal if respiration stops or the heart rate slows down.

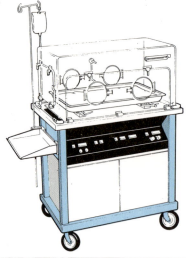

Examination of the newborn

Once breathing has been established, the doctor will examine the baby and the length and head circumference will be measured. In this initial examination he will look for any congenital abnormalities, and assess how the birth has affected the baby.

Approximately one or two per cent of babies have some congenital abnormality. A few of them must be treated urgently, whilst more require only minor treatment at a later stage. Some require no treatment at all. Particular attention is paid to the palate, heart, back, hips, and genitalia, as these are the common sites of congenital abnormalities.

Few babies are badly affected by birth, but after a difficult or prolonged delivery there may be excessive bruising or other signs indicating birth trauma. Both undue sleepiness and excessive activity during the first few days can be signs of a difficult delivery, and the baby may need very gentle handling. A further examination of the baby is usually performed at about one week, or before discharge from hospital. The doctor will be interested in checking for problems such as feeding difficulties, infections, jaundice, heart murmurs or unstable hips. This examination should be seen as the first of many routine health assessments to be made throughout childhood by a doctor or community child health doctor.

Feeding difficulties

Some delay in establishing satisfactory feeding in the first few days is very common and not usually serious. The difficulties can result merely from the inexperience of the baby and mother, and advice from a midwife or nurse may be all that is required. Such counselling is particularly important with breast-feeding, where specific advice on the care of the nipples and breasts, and reassurance about adequacy of milk production is necessary.

After a difficult delivery a baby may be sleepy and show little interest in feeding for a few days. However if a previously eager baby loses interest in feeding this suggests the onset of an infection or some other problem, and the doctor should be consulted.

Unstable and clicking hips

The hips of all newborn babies should be examined on several occasions. A few babies are born with the hip joint dislocated or unstable. Provided this abnormality is recognized early, treatment is relatively simple, consisting of temporary splinting or immobilizing in plaster. If not detected in infancy, surgery may be needed to correct the abnormality.

A large number of babies have hips that make a click when they are examined. Most hips that click are otherwise perfectly normal, but these babies may need medical follow-up until it is certain that no hip disease is present.

Infections in the newborn period

Newborn babies catch infections easily because their body defences are immature. Scrupulous cleanliness is necessary in the nursery, and people who may be carrying an infection should not handle babies.

Some infections will be obvious, such as sticky eye or septic spots on the skin. However a baby who is generally off colour, or otherwise unwell, could be suffering from an infection. The doctor will find out by taking swabs from the nose, throat and navel. Stool and urine specimens may also be collected. The samples are sent to a laboratory to see if any infection is present. If an infection is found, or one is suspected, the doctor will usually start antibiotic treatment.

Low birth weight babies

There are two main reasons why some babies are very small at birth. They are either born before they are due, or they have not grown sufficiently in the womb. Babies born early are called 'preterm' and babies who have grown poorly are called 'small-for-dates'. Until quite recently all babies who weighed less than 5½lb (2.5kg) at birth were called 'premature' but this term is gradually being replaced by 'low birth weight'.

Some small babies are in fact genetically small. Their size relates to the size of their parents rather than to pregnancy complications. Such babies are otherwise healthy at birth.

Preterm babies. Babies are born early either because the mother goes into labour spontaneously, or because labour is induced early by the obstetrician, a doctor who specializes in childbirth.

The spontaneous early onset of labour often occurs because the mother is suffering from a pregnancy complication such as toxaemia (also known as pre-eclampsia) and has high blood pressure and fluid retention.

Obstetricians induce early labour if they are concerned about the health of the baby or the mother. This can be because of high blood pressure in the mother, some other illness or pregnancy complication, or because tests have shown that the foetus is not growing normally.

Small-for-dates babies. In the womb the foetus receives all the necessary nutrients from the mother by way of the placenta. Provided the mother is eating normally, her diet will not affect the baby's size. However, if the placenta is malfunctioning the foetus will not receive adequate nutrition and this leads to poor growth and weight gain. Placental insufficiency is more common in mothers who smoke heavily, and it may occur in twin pregnancy or with mothers who have high blood pressure or other pregnancy complications. Sometimes no cause is found. Many of the factors which lead to problems with the placenta are also associated with early labour. Low birth weight babies are often both early and small.

Breathing problems
Many babies born four weeks or more before they are due develop some difficulty with breathing and this may become severe. Respiratory distress syndrome (RDS) occurs because immature lungs do not remain inflated after their initial expansion with the first breath. As a result the work of breathing is increased and exhaustion of the respiratory muscles can easily occur.

If the RDS is mild, the air in the incubator is enriched with oxygen for the baby to breathe. If higher concentrations of oxygen are needed a special oxygen hood (or head box) is fitted over the baby's head. With severe RDS these measures may not be enough, and the baby is then connected to a ventilator which takes over the work of breathing. While babies with RDS are being given oxygen they need frequent blood tests to ensure that the right amount of oxygen is being given, as both too little or too much may be harmful.

Some low birth weight babies have episodes (known as apnoeic attacks) in which they stop breathing. These are due to the respiratory centre in the brain, which controls regular breathing, not being fully operational because of the baby's immaturity.

The machines that monitor the baby's respiration have an alarm that sounds if the baby stops breathing, alerting the nurses to the need to start the baby's breathing again.

Low blood glucose
It is important that the level of glucose in the blood does not fall too low as it provides the source of energy for all the vital body functions. The body can normally maintain the blood glucose level between meals by releasing glucose from special stores in the liver. Carbohydrate in the diet is converted to glucose in the body and the liver stores are replenished at meal times.

In low birth weight babies, particularly in those who are small-for-dates due to poor nutrition from the placenta, the liver stores of glucose are small and may not be enough to maintain the blood glucose. If the level drops too low the baby may have episodes of apnoea or develop convulsions.

To prevent this happening, low birth weight babies are given frequent feeds or glucose drinks shortly after birth, or are given a glucose drip into a vein. Additionally, frequent blood tests to measure blood glucose are done in the first few days.

Jaundice
Many babies have mild jaundice in the first week of life. Once babies are born they do not need as many red cells as were needed in the womb, and the excess blood cells are broken down in the body, forming a yellow waste product called bilirubin. This bilirubin in the circulation gives the yellow colouring in the skin and other tissues, which we call jaundice.

Excess bilirubin is removed by the liver, but in preterm infants the liver may not be sufficiently developed. This leads to poor excretion of bilirubin, resulting in more marked jaundice. Severe jaundice may lead to brain damage, so that if a newborn baby is becoming even moderately jaundiced the doctor will order tests to check the blood level of bilirubin. If it approaches dangerous levels corrective treatment is started.

Phototherapy may be the only treatment necessary to alleviate jaundice. The baby lies naked, with eyes covered, under a fluorescent light. If treatment with phototherapy is not enough, the doctor may do an exchange blood transfusion.

Parental reaction
Inevitably parental reactions to a low birth weight baby are mixed. They may include disappointment, anxiety, and feelings of rejection. Many parents initially find it difficult to feel any attraction or love for a very small and scrawny baby and may feel guilty and angry. There is nothing shameful about any of these reactions and in a good special care baby unit they will be acknowledged and understood, and there will be opportunities for talking them through with the staff.

In addition, pregnancy and delivery may not have been straightforward, and may have included the baby arriving before all preparations were made, the mother being rushed into hospital unexpectedly, or kept in hospital for a long time. The delivery may have been induced and a forceps delivery is usual because of the small size of the baby.

Furthermore there may be serious anxieties over the health of the baby. He may be too small to hold or cuddle, and need to be removed to the unfamiliar and perhaps intimidating surroundings of a special care baby unit.

Parents should try and see their baby in the special care baby unit as often as possible, and should do as much caring for him as possible. Obviously if he is very small and sick he may have to be largely cared for by the doctors and nurses, but parents can still come and touch him and hold his hand. This contact is important for the parents and is important also for the baby. Parents are the people a baby needs most of all and getting to know them starts immediately after birth.

Breast feeding

There is no doubt that breast feeding is the ideal for nearly all babies in the first few months of life. Even if it is not satisfactory and a change has to be made to bottle feeding, it is well worth trying as even a short period on the breast will benefit the baby (see right). However it does suit some mothers better to bottle feed and with modern modified baby milks bottle feeding is perfectly satisfactory provided the manufacturers' instructions are followed in preparation and the mother pays scrupulous attention to hygiene.

The first week of breast feeding
A baby can suck strongly immediately after birth and can be put to the breast straight away. It is important to realize however that it is not always easy to build up a feeding relationship. It can sometimes take at least three weeks to settle into a routine. For the first three days the breasts produce a special secretion called colostrum which protects

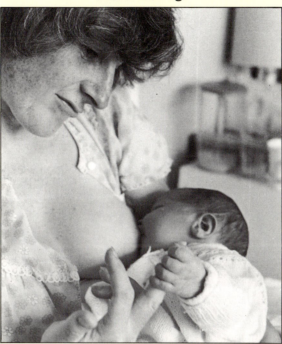

the baby from early infection. On about the fourth day the breasts start producing milk. This is often a particularly difficult time for both mothers and

babies. Mothers' breasts and nipples may feel sore and feeds can seem endless and erratic. This difficult stage does pass, and a routine is established.

Benefits of breast feeding
1. Breast milk contains all the necessary nourishment for a baby. Unlike cow's milk, nothing needs to be added or taken away.

2. Breast milk is easily digestible and so the baby is unlikely to suffer from constipation or indigestion.

3. A breast-fed baby is less likely to suffer from tummy upset or diarrhoea.

4. Breast milk contains proteins which confer some immunity against infection.

5. Liability to eczema and asthma is reduced.

6. The mother has more time to rest or play with her baby as she does not have to bother mixing feeds or sterilizing bottles.

7. Breast feeding provides the baby with the necessary emotional security and helps to form an important bond between the mother and baby.

Feeding comfort

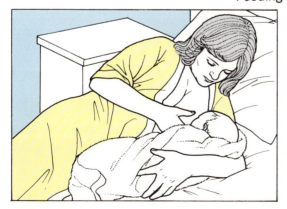
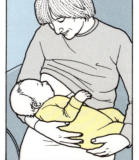
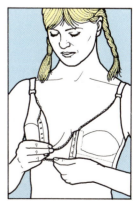

Women choose a variety of positions in which to breast feed their babies. Most sit comfortably in an armchair (middle), but some women prefer to breast feed lying down (left).

A firm supporting bra is essential and it helps to have one which is adjustable in size to allow for breasts changing shape. The

bra (right) fastens at the front and one breast can be exposed at a time by unbuttoning a flap.

Inherited diseases and congenital abnormalities

INHERITED CHARACTERISTICS ARE PASSED from parent to child at the time of conception. Within the sperm and the egg are a set of chromosomes derived from the parents, each built up of hundreds of genes. Genes are the basic units of inheritance. At fertilization these two sets of chromosomes come together and influence the future development of a new individual.

For each inherited characteristic there is a pair of genes, one from the father and one from the mother. Often these genes are identical but sometimes they will be different. If one gene of one pair has a major effect on the development of the individual it is said to be a dominant gene. Genes of small effect are said to be recessive, and their effect is only noted when both of the gene pair are recessive genes. Many individual characteristics, such as skin and eye colour, height, intelligence and appearance, have an inherited component. There are also some diseases which are due to inherited factors.

The genes causing inherited disease may be dominant or recessive. With dominant disorders only one of a pair of genes needs to be abnormal for the disease to be manifest, so the condition can be passed on by an affected parent even when the other parent is healthy. On average, half of the children of such a mating will inherit the harmful genes and the disease.

In the case of diseases due to recessive genes, an individual has to inherit an abnormal gene from each parent for the disease to be manifest. Although the parents will be carriers of the harmful gene they are unlikely to know this, as the effect of the gene is neutralized by a dominant normal gene. If both parents are carriers of the same harmful recessive gene, then on average one in four of the children of the marriage will manifest the disease. The chances of healthy unrelated persons carrying the same harmful gene is fortunately small. Cousin marriages and other marriages between relatives have a higher risk.

Sex-linked inheritance is a special type of recessive inheritance in which females who carry the harmful gene have no features of the disease, but on average half of their sons will have the condition. Daughters do not have the disease, but half are carriers of the condition.

Genetic disorders are not necessarily obvious at birth or in infancy. They may reveal themslves at various stages, depending on the disorder. The following are examples of inherited diseases. There are over 1,000 different diseases known to be inherited; most of them are uncommon or rare.

> **Dominant conditions:** achondroplasia, familial hypercholesterolaemia, Friedrich's ataxia, hereditary spherocytosis, Huntingdon's chorea, neurofibromatosis.
>
> **Recessive conditions:** cystic fibrosis, galactosaemia, phenylketonuria, sickle cell disease, Tay Sachs disease, thalassaemia.
>
> **Sex linked conditions:** Christmas disease, colour blindness, haemophilia, muscular dystrophy (Duchenne type).

Other hereditary diseases

There are other diseases which commonly run in families, and are not inherited in the manner described

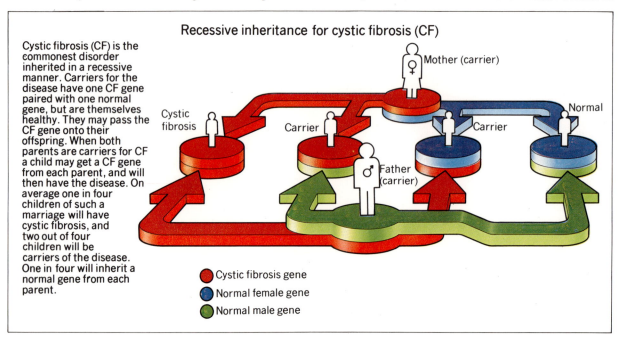

Recessive inheritance for cystic fibrosis (CF)

Cystic fibrosis (CF) is the commonest disorder inherited in a recessive manner. Carriers for the disease have one CF gene paired with one normal gene, but are themselves healthy. They may pass the CF gene onto their offspring. When both parents are carriers for CF a child may get a CF gene from each parent, and will then have the disease. On average one in four children of such a marriage will have cystic fibrosis, and two out of four children will be carriers of the disease. One in four will inherit a normal gene from each parent.

Mother (carrier)

Cystic fibrosis

Carrier

Carrier

Normal

Father (carrier)

● Cystic fibrosis gene
● Normal female gene
● Normal male gene

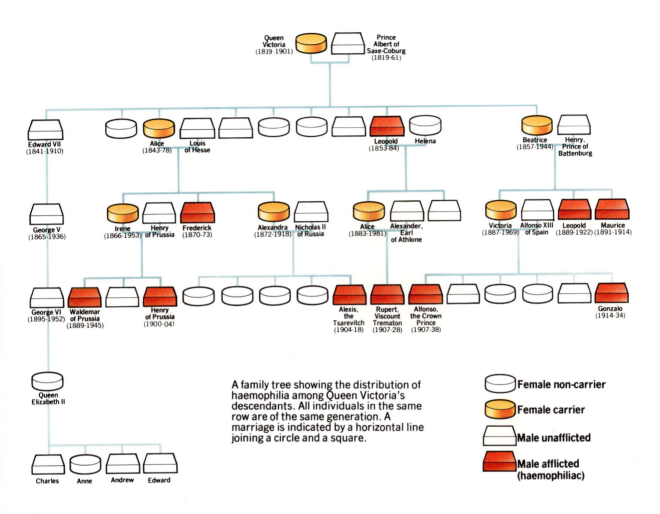

A family tree showing the distribution of haemophilia among Queen Victoria's descendants. All individuals in the same row are of the same generation. A marriage is indicated by a horizontal line joining a circle and a square.

- Female non-carrier
- Female carrier
- Male unafflicted
- Male afflicted (haemophiliac)

Chromosomes in Down's Syndrome

Chromosomes are small thread like structures occurring in the nucleus of each cell in the body. They carry all the genetic material which determines the inherited characteristics of the individual. Using special techniques the chromosomes can be identified and counted. Normal individuals have 46 chromosomes arranged in pairs. Down's syndrome (Mongolism) is due to each cell having an extra bit of chromosomal material — usually a whole extra chromosome (circle on diagram). This is called a chromosomal trisomy.

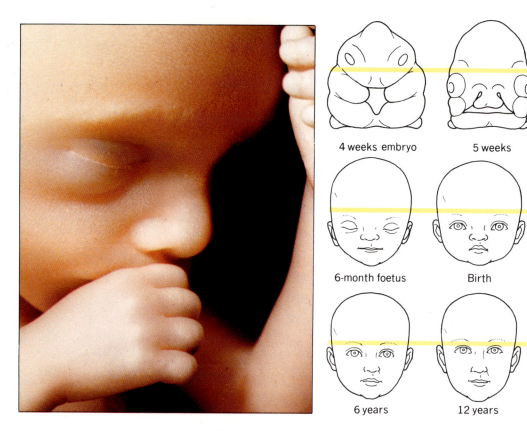

4 weeks embryo	5 weeks	8 weeks
6-month foetus	Birth	Infancy
6 years	12 years	Adult

above involving a single pair of genes. For many of these conditions there is a genetic predisposition (conferred on an individual by several pairs of genes) which leads to the disease if other environmental factors are also present. This type of inheritance is known as polygenic inheritance, as several pairs of genes are inolved. Conditions resulting from polygenic inheritance are: cleft palate, diabetes (some cases), hare lip, Hirshprungs disease, pyloric stenosis, spina bifida.

Chromosomal disorders

Genetic disorders involve either one pair of genes, or in polygenic inheritance only a few genes. The genes are carried on chromosomes, each chromosome having hundreds or thousands of genes. The normal individual has 23 pairs of chromosomes, one for each pair coming from the mother, and one from the father.

Occasionally errors in cell division in forming the sperm or the ovum may lead to individuals with too much, or too little, chromosomal material. For instance, Down's syndrome (mongolism) is due to every cell in the body having either one extra chromosome, or an extra part of a chromosome.

Most chromosomal disorders are not compatible with life, and either lead to miscarriage in pregnancy, or death of the child soon after birth. In a few

chromosomal disorders, of which Down's syndrome is the most common, prolonged survival can occur. Some chromosomal abnormalities can recur in families, and in each case individual genetic counselling is needed.

Congenital abnormalities

Congenital abnormalities are structural defects of the body present at birth. Many may be immediately apparent, such as hare lip or spina bifida, but if the defect is internal it may only be detected later, for example congenital heart disease and congenital dislocation of the hip.

Congenital abnormalities may be inherited, or may be due to something going wrong at conception, or during development. We know, for example, that exposure of a pregnant woman to rubella infection, or to certain drugs and toxins, can lead to congenital abnormalities. Irradiation from Xrays, nutritional deficiencies, and other hazards may lead to major or minor abnormalities, and in many cases no cause has yet been found for the defect. More than one factor may be involved. It is now thought that spina bifida may be due to the combination of genetic predisposition and maternal vitamin deficiency around the time of conception or in early pregnancy.

If a couple have a child with a congenital malforma-

Development of the face In the embryo the face is formed by the development of separate parts which go on to form the nose, and the upper and lower jaws (top row, left). At a slightly later stage these separate parts join together to give the complete face. The face goes on developing and changing shape throughout childhood (left). It can be seen from the diagram that in early childhood the eyes are below the midline of the face, but as the child grows the face becomes longer due to growth of bony sinuses in the cheeks and the eyes gradually 'move up' in relation to the midline of the face.

Sometimes the joining of the separate parts in embryonic life is not complete, and a hare lip and/or a cleft palate may result.

The picture (far left) shows a foetus at five months, sucking his thumb.

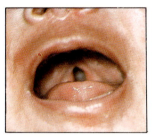

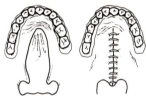

Cleft Palate Developmental clefts may involve the lips, the gums and the palate, and are of varying severity. A cleft palate (top) can interfere with feeding in infancy as the baby cannot suck properly.

It also interferes with speech, so needs to be surgically repaired (shown above) during the first year of life, before the baby starts learning to talk.

Cousin marriage

The way in which recessive disorders are inherited is if both parents are carriers of some harmful gene, although they themselves are healthy. On average, one in four of their children will inherit the harmful gene from each parent and manifest the disease.

For most recessive disorders, being a carrier of the disease is uncommon, so the risk of two unrelated individuals both carrying the same harmful gene is small. With a related couple, however, they will have some identical genes, and therefore the risks of having a child with a recessive disorder are higher than for unrelated people.

With marriages between first cousins, where there is no family history of inherited disease, this risk is not great, and in many societies cousin marriages are common. Genetic counsellors are happy to advise related couples who are thinking of having children on the extent of the risk involved.

tion they may want to talk over the possibility of the malformation recurring again in other children they may have. A paediatrician or specialist genetic counsellor will be able to advise.

Genetic counselling

Information and help given to people concerned about the risk of inherited disease is known as genetic counselling. It is beneficial to couples who already have a child with a serious disease or a congenital abnormality, those with a family history of inherited disease, and those who are marrying, or are married to, first cousins or other relatives.

Before any advice can be given the genetic counsellor will need to have a precise diagnosis, wherever possible, of any affected individuals in the family. He may want to have general information on other members of the family including any who died in infancy or childhood.

The discussion will include an estimate of the risk of having an abnormal baby. For some conditions with known mode of inheritance, the risks can be determined accurately, but in other situations they may be less precise. These risks need to be considered in relation to the risks that every couple face when they have a baby; one to two per cent of children are stillborn or die in the newborn period, and one to two per cent have significant congenital abnormality.

With some inherited diseases it is possible to determine whether individuals are carriers of a harmful recessive or sex-linked gene. These include sickle cell disease, thalassaemia, Tay Sachs disease, haemophilia, and muscular dystrophy.

Knowledge of the possible risks of having a child with an inherited condition is not enough; some knowledge of the severity of the condition is also needed. Many familial conditions can be treated (for example, pyloric stenosis or hare lip) and are therefore unlikely to deter a couple from having children, while others may cause considerable disability.

For some conditions AMNIOCENTESIS in early pregnancy will enable doctors to say whether or not the foetus is affected by a familial disorder or chromosome abnormality. The counsellor will help the couple to consider whether an abortion would be acceptable to them in the event of a serious abnormality being diagnosed early in pregnancy.

It is often appropriate to encourage each partner to express personal feelings about family life with or without an affected child. Genetic counselling is always individualized because each situation is unique. The counsellor will not only have technical knowledge but will also be sensitive to the needs and worries of those who seek advice. The counsellor's aim is to inform, and to help a couple make their own decisions.

Infectious diseases

INFECTIOUS DISEASES ARE EXTREMELY common in childhood. An infection starts when certain microorganisms invade the body and start to multiply. The body in turn reacts to this and tries to fight off the infection. The illness which results is partly due to the effects of the multiplying microorganisms and partly due to the body's reactions.

Many types of microorganisms live in the human body without causing disease but those which do make people ill are called 'pathogenic'. The most common pathogenic microorganisms are bacteria and viruses. Antibiotics can be used to stop bacteria reproducing, but most viruses cannot be destroyed by antibiotics and it is usually necessary in viral diseases to wait until the infection is overcome by the body's own immune system.

Bacteria can usually be seen and indentified under a microscope in a laboratory. Virus particles are generally too small to be seen under an ordinary microscope and techniques for identifying them can take several weeks.

Infectious diseases are contagious and spread from person to person in various ways, by coughing, sneezing, direct contact, or contact with vomit, urine or faeces.

Incubation period
Some infectious diseases have a latent period between the time the infection first invades the body and the time of the onset of symptoms. This is called the incubation period (see charts over page).

Quarantine period
The quarantine period is the time in which a person with a specific infection is capable of transferring that infection to other people. Hygiene, isolation during quarantine periods and immunization are important ways of preventing the spread of infection (see charts over page).

Infectious diseases Infections can be caused by bacteria, by viruses, and by other microorganisms. The infection may be localized to one part of the body, or more widespread with manifestations in many systems. Common sites and features of infections are shown in this diagram.

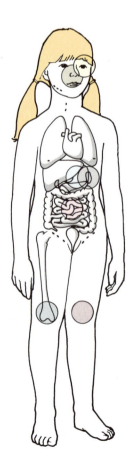

Tonsils and adenoids In young children sore throats due to infection are common. Enlargement of the tonsils and adenoids may occur, and infection can spread to the ears.

The stomach Infections of the stomach due to eating infected food gives rise to vomiting, and maybe abdominal pain.

The bones Infection of bones is uncommon, but infection may spread to the bones via the blood stream giving rise to osteomyelitis.

Eyes Redness of the eyes, with watering and sometimes sticky pus, indicates infection, and is known as conjunctivitis. Although often due to localized bacterial infection, conjunctivitis may be due to measles and other generalized infections.

The spleen The spleen is part of the body's immune defence system. It may become enlarged with infectious disease.

The intestines Infection of the intestines due to eating contaminated food gives rise to diarrhoea and colicky abdominal pain. Severe abdominal pain may indicate localized infections, as occurs with appendicitis.

The skin The skin helps to protect the body from infection. However it may become locally infected, as with boils and impetigo. It may also show rashes indicating more generalized infection.

Hygiene for newborn babies

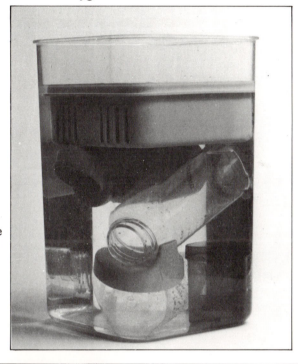

Small babies are susceptible to infections as the body defence mechanisms that give protection are not fully developed. It is therefore essential that attention is paid to cleanliness.

Breast-fed babies are less likely to develop infections, especially gastroenteritis, than babies who are bottle fed. Bottle feeding, however, is perfectly satisfactory providing scrupulous attention is paid to hygiene when feeding and using feeding bottles.

Another factor is keeping the skin clean. The napkin area can readily become sore if there is prolonged contact with urine, and this can precipitate skin infection, causing bacteria or thrush. Regular cleaning of the skin, and using a barrier cream, is helpful. Washing the face and eyes is important, and helps to protect against infections such as sticky eyes.

If you are going to look after your baby well, these simple rules should become second nature to you.
1. Always wash your hands before preparing a baby's feed.
2. Follow the instructions given for the feed. Do not give extra milk powder to make the feed a bit stronger.
3. Bottles and teats should be washed out after use, and then kept in sterilizing fluid (see left).
4. If you make up a whole day's feed together, keep it in a refrigerator. Never keep feeds warm for long periods — it promotes the growth of bacteria which could cause gastroenteritis.
5. Never give your baby milk that has been prepared for longer than about 24 hours.
6. Keep your baby away from people with infections, however trivial they may seem. If the infection is passed on to the baby it could be serious.

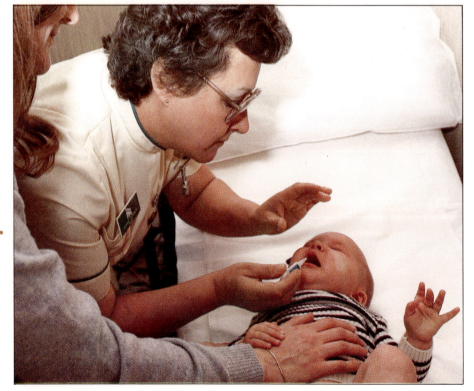

Immunization protects children against whooping cough, diphtheria, polio, measles and tetanus. It is very rare for an immunized child to catch one of these diseases, but if they do, the attack will be much milder and less dangerous than if the child had not been immunized.

The vaccines which immunize against whooping cough, diphtheria and tetanus are usually combined into one 'triple' vaccine which is given by injection. Polio vaccine is given by mouth (see left), usually at the same time as the 'triple' vaccine.

You should take your baby for the first series of immunizations at about three months. The second is usually given at about six months and the third before the child is a year old. The timetable (see page 48) does vary slightly, so check with your doctor.

Immunization

IMMUNIZATION PROCEDURES DEVELOP the body's resistance to specific infections. This is achieved by either giving a live, but modified, infectious agent to induce a very mild infection (polio, measles and BCG immunization) or by injecting killed microorganisms or their products (diptheria, pertussis, tetanus).

The bottom table opposite lists the incubation and quarantine periods of common infectious diseases. Some can be prevented by prior immunization. The commonly recommended immunizations of childhood are given in the top table opposite. All healthy children should be fully immunized to prevent them developing these preventable and potentially serious conditions. If your child has any other disease you should discuss with your doctor whether immunization is appropriate.

If you are going abroad, especially to tropical or sub-tropical regions, you and your child run the risk of catching dangerous infections and diseases. You should consult your doctor to find out which vaccinations you need (see table below).

Going Abroad				
Disease	Risk Areas	Vaccination	Period of cover	Reactions/notes
Yellow fever	Africa, Central and South America	1 injection at least 10 days before going abroad. Must be 2-week gap between this and polio.	From 10 days after injection, for 10 years	Caution if allergic to eggs. Not given to children under 1 year old, or to pregnant women. Certificate needed.
Cholera	Africa, Asia, Middle East	2 injections, 1 to 4 weeks apart	6 days after injection for 6 months	Certificate needed. NB Take care over hygiene as additional precaution.
Polio	Everywhere, except Australia, New New Zealand, Northern Europe, North America	Oral drops 3 doses, 4-8 weeks apart	Immediately after 3rd injection, for 3 years	
Typhoid		2 injections, 4-6 weeks apart	After 2nd injection, for 3 years	
Tetanus	Everywhere	Course of 3 injections initially, then booster injection if at risk	Immediately, for 5 years	
Infectious hepatitis	Places where sanitation is primitive	No specific vaccine. 1 injection of immuno-globulin if in high risk area	Immediately, for 4-6 months	Take care over hygiene as additional precaution.

Malaria
Anti-malaria tablets are available and must be taken if you are visiting Africa (particularly Central Africa), areas of Central and South America, South-East Asia and parts of the Middle East. Ask your doctor for details.

Take the tablets before, during and for a month after your visit (even if you are only stopping over in one of these countries).

Rabies
It is a serious hazard all over the world, including parts of Europe. You can contract rabies if bitten, scratched or even licked by an infected animal (dog, cat, fox).

Be extremely careful, particularly where children are concerned. If they are bitten or scratched get medical attention immediately.

Smallpox
It has been accepted by the World Health Organization that the disease has been erradicated, but vaccination may still be required for travellers to some countries. Check with your doctor.

Hygiene
Observe the following precautions when travelling abroad:

1. Wash your own, and your child's, hands thoroughly before eating.
2. Make sure that drinking water is safe.
3. Be cautious about eating raw vegetables, unpeeled fruit, ice-cream, ice cubes, raw shellfish, underdone meat and fish, and reheated food.

Vaccination and Immunization Procedures

Age	Vaccine	Method	Notes
2-3 months	Triple immunization: DTP = diphtheria, tetanus & pertussis (whooping cough)	injection	
	Poliomyelitis	drops by mouth	
5-6 months	DTP	injection	
	Poliomyelitis	drops by mouth	
9-11 months	DTP	injection	
2nd year of life	Measles	injection	
4-6 years school or nursery school entry	DT	injection	Preferably 3 years after basic course.
	Poliomyelitis — booster	drops by mouth	
10-14 years	TB/BCG vac. Rubella vac. (girls only)		If skin test negative. All girls of this age should be given rubella vac., regardless of whether they have had German measles or not.
15-18 years school leaving age	Poliomyelitis vac.	drops by mouth	
	Tetanus booster	injection	

Incubation Periods

Disease	Interval between exposure to infection & developing symptoms	Contagious period
Bacillary dysentery	1-7 days	Until bacteriological tests are clear.
Chickenpox	11-21 days	24 hours before spots erupt until scabs form about 6 days later.
Food poisoning	2-24 hours, depending on the causative microorganism	variable.
German measles (rubella)	14-21 days	From a few days before to 4 days after onset.
Infectious jaundice (hepatitis)	Between 15 and 50 days, commonly 28	From a few days before to 7 days after onset.
Measles	10-15 days	Few days before to 5 days after rash appears.
Mumps	12-26 days	From a few days before symptoms until swelling has subsided.
Scarlet fever	2-5 days	Until antibiotic treatment is started.
Tuberculosis	4-6 weeks	Only infectious in some cases.
Whooping cough	7-10 days	From 7 days after exposure to 21 days after onset of cough.

Infectious diarrhoea

THE SUDDEN ONSET of diarrhoea in childhood is usually due to infection. When the diarrhoea is accompanied by vomiting, the infection is referred to as gastroenteritis, and may be due to bacterial or viral infection of the digestive system. In young children diarrhoea and vomiting sometimes occur with infection elsewhere, such as tonsillitis or urinary infection. Dysentery is a bacterial infection of the bowel characterized by severe diarrhoea with little or no vomiting.

Diarrhoea has a short incubation period of one or two days, and because it is highly infectious several members of the family may be affected at the same time. The severity of the illness will vary, from only one or two loose stools to so many fluid motions that the child becomes severely dehydrated through loss of fluid. In dysentery the stools often contain mucus and flecks of blood.

Vomiting is a frequent accompaniment to diarrhoea in childhood, and under the age of two years, vomiting and diarrhoea together can rapidly lead to serious dehydration. In dehydration the mouth feels dry, often the eyes appear sunken, and the circulation becomes weak because of the lack of fluid. If this occurs, consult a doctor at once. Dehydration needs urgent treatment, preferably in hospital.

Abdominal pain may accompany gastroenteritis. It is not usually severe, although in dysentery there can be waves of griping abdominal pain. Continuous abdominal pain is unlikely to be due to infectious diarrhoea. Slight fever occurs occasionally with gastroenteritis, and more commonly with dysentery.

When examining children suffering from diarrhoea the doctor's main concern will be in assessing whether or not the child's body is becoming dehydrated from loss of fluid. Doctors may also arrange for a stool specimen to be sent to a laboratory so that the infection can be identified.

Treatment for diarrhoea is directed towards preventing and correcting dehydration, the relief of symptoms, and the prevention of the spread of infection to others. If the child is not dehydrated, or only mildly so, it may be possible to give fluid by mouth. Even if the child has been vomiting previously, by giving him frequent small drinks of clear fluid containing glucose and salts, it is often possible to maintain the fluid balance in the body. A suitable drink is obtainable from pharmacists or can be prescribed by the doctor. It is a solution of sodium chloride and glucose powder which comes in sachets ready for preparation, and is specially formulated.

If the child is dehydrated when first seen, or continues to vomit fluid, then an intravenous drip (carrying fluid from a bag, via a small tube, into a vein) is

Treatment of diarrhoea in babies

Diarrhoea is a frequency of loose or watery stools. Different kinds of infection can lead to this condition in childhood. Diarrhoea can be very serious, especially when it is combined with vomiting, as it can lead to severe dehydration. This is particularly the case with babies under two years whose bodies are unable to stand much fluid loss. A baby with diarrhoea should be given plenty of liquid to drink in order to maintain the fluid balance of the body. Frequent small drinks of cooled, boiled water containing glucose and salt or a suitable drink obtainable either on prescription from the doctor or from the chemist should be provided. If the baby is unable to take in fluid by mouth or is already dehydrated, he will need to be taken into hospital urgently and put on an intravenous drip. For children over two the risk of dehydration applies,

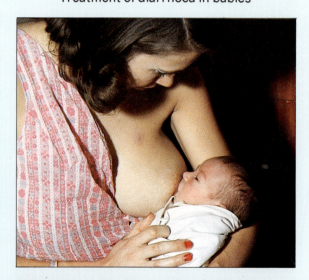

but is less likely. However it is still important that they are given plenty of fluids. Medicine such as preparations of kaolin can also be given to soothe the intestines and treat the diarrhoea. However if the

child is unable to retain any fluid the doctor should be called immediately. Careful hygiene is essential in all cases in order to prevent the spread of infection.

Infectious diarrhoea and gastroenteritis are very uncommon in breast-fed babies(left). Because breast milk goes straight from mother to child it cannot become contaminated by microorganisms from outside. Breast milk also contains proteins which confer some immunity against infection.

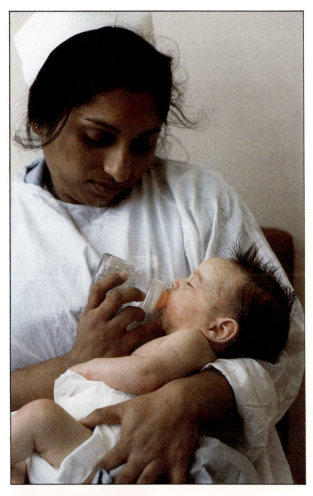

necessary. The child will need to be taken to a hospital urgently and admitted to the infectious diseases unit or the children's department.

The diarrhoea seldom persists for more than a few hours after treatment with special drinks or with intravenous fluid. Occasionally it may recur as the child is put back onto mild or solid food. Infectious diarrhoea often lasts for only 24 hours and is seldom prolonged. The prevention and treatment of dehydration are of prime importance, but the diarrhoea itself may be treated medicinally. Preparations of kaolin are most widely used and soothe the intestines as well as alleviating the diarrhoea. Antibiotics are not usually given for acute diarrhoea, even though many of them are due to bacterial infections. They do not shorten the attack, and they may, in fact, prolong the period the child continues to be a carrier of the infection.

Prevention of spread of infection to others involves careful hygiene, remembering that stools and vomit may be infected. As far as possible the child should be isolated and preferably should use a separate toilet. Hands should be washed extra carefully after using the toilet. Soiled clothes may carry infection, and should be promptly laundered. If a stool specimen shows the infection was due to dysentry organisms the health department will advise on measures to be taken.

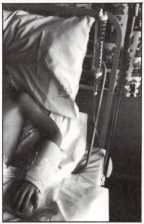

drip. A tube attached to a bag filled with fluid is inserted into one of the child's veins (left). In this way the child is provided with the necessary fluid. The baby (top) is receiving a clear feed. Cooled, boiled water with a level teaspoonful of sugar and a half a teaspoonful of salt in each pint is substituted for the baby's usual feed for 24 hours. On the second day the baby should be given his usual formula diluted to half the strength.

Intravenous drip and clear feed If a child becomes dehydrated or continues to vomit then he will need to be taken to hospital urgently and put on an intravenous

Summary

1. Diarrhoea is highly infectious.

2. It has a short incubation period of one or two days.

3. Diarrhoea seldom lasts for more than a few days once appropriate treatment has been given.

4. Diarrhoea is dangerous because it can lead to severe dehydration, especially in babies under two and when it is combined with vomiting. Dehydration needs urgent treatment so a doctor should be consulted immediately.

Serious features

1. When it occurs in young infants.

2. Very frequent watery motions.

3. Pus or blood in the stools (possibly dysentry).

4. Fever of 101°F/38°C or more.

5. Sunken eyes, which is a sign of dehydration.

6. Recurrent vomiting.

Consult a doctor without delay.

Measles

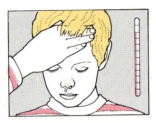

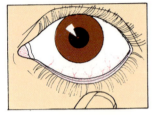

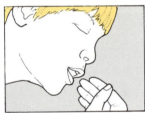

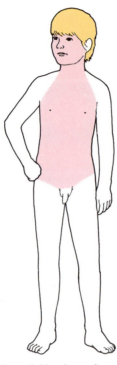

MEASLES IS A HIGHLY infectious viral illness, which non-immunized children usually get in early childhood. It is characterized by high fever and a rash and may be severe. One attack gives permanent immunity. The incubation period is 10 to 12 days from the time of contact to the onset of symptoms, and about 14 days to the onset of the rash. The child can infect others from the time of onset of the first symptoms until about five days after the rash has started to come out.

There is a period of three to four days before the rash appears during which the child becomes more ill with a runny nose and raised temperature. There is a lot of nasal catarrh and this is often blood-stained. The temperature gradually increases over this period, up to about 101°F (39°C) but it can go higher. There is a dry cough which accompanies the catarrh and fever, and the eyes become red with conjunctivitis.

For a day or two before the rash starts there are spots in the mouth, and on the inside of the cheeks. The rash usually starts on the fourth day. The more extensive and pronounced it is, the more severely ill the child will be. With the onset of the rash the child becomes more ill with a high fever, up to 105°F/41°C, and a worsening cough for one or two days. When the rash starts to fade, the temperature rapidly returns to normal. Over the next week the skin may have a brownish discolouration and be flakey, but this soon clears too.

Measles may be complicated by a secondary infection of the ears or lungs, but this is uncommon in children who were well before the onset of the infection.

There is no specific treatment for measles. The child can be given paracetamol or soluble aspirin for the high temperature, and a linctus to help soothe the cough. The child will probably want to remain in bed while he is ill, and should be given plenty of fluid to drink.

Symptoms Measles can be unpleasant since it involves the child having the symptoms of a severe, feverish cold even before a rash has appeared. As the fever worsens over the first few days of the illness, a dry cough develops with a runny nose. This nasal catarrh may be bloodstained. The eyes become red and irritated with conjunctivitis. After these cold symptoms have continued for two days white spots appear inside the mouth — this is a definite indication that the child has measles. On about the fourth day the rash appears and the fever and cough become more severe. A few days later all symptoms will begin to fade.

Kopliks spots (right) These spots are the surest indication that a child has measles and the doctor will look for them when diagnosing the illness. They break out in the mouth, on the inside of the cheek and around the back teeth. The spots have tiny white centres, surrounded by redness. They usually appear two days after the symptoms have begun, and two days after they appear the rash breaks out (far right).

The rash Measles rash consists of dark pink spots which merge to form blotches. It occurs first behind the ears and across the forehead on about the fourth day of the illness. It will spread to the front and back of the trunk and then finally to the limbs where the rash will be less dense.

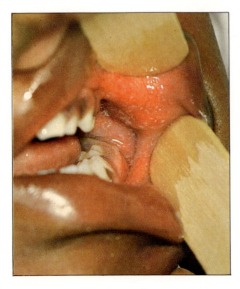

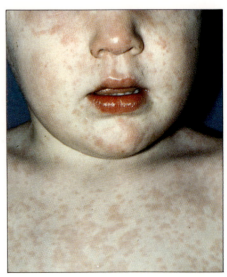

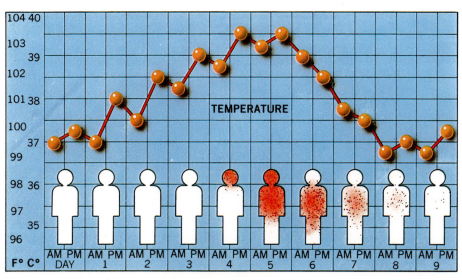

	104 40											
	103											
	39											
	102											
	101 38					**TEMPERATURE**						
	100											
	37											
	99											

F° C° AM PM / AM PM / AM PM / AM PM / AM PM / AM PM / AM PM / AM PM / AM PM / AM PM
DAY 1 2 3 4 5 6 7 8 9

Temperature chart This chart shows the normal variation of body temperature during a bout of measles. Day one represents the day on which the cold symptoms first occur. The variation in the rash is also shown, as it coincides with the fever. The rash usually breaks out on the fourth day and the temperature will then be quite high, and could go even higher the next day as the rash extends to the body. As the temperature drops on the sixth and seventh day, the rash will start to fade.

Summary

1. Measles is a virus which is highly contagious. It is transmitted through droplets from the nose and throat of an infected person.

2. The period between contracting the infection and the symptoms appearing is from seven to fourteen days; usually ten days.

3. Fever with a dry cough, red eyes and runny nose. On the second or third day white spots appear in the mouth. On the fourth day a rash breaks out and the fever is high. The rash spreads for several days, then all symptoms subside.

4. Keep the child comfortable with plenty to drink.

5. Live measles vaccine is given in infancy and is effective for many years.

Immunization Treatment Complications

Immunization It is usual to have children vaccinated against measles in infancy (see Immunization chart page 48). Up to five per cent of vaccinated children do later contract the disease but usually only in a mild form.
Gammaglobulin Measles can be prevented, or made milder, if a child is given gammaglobulin before the symptoms appear. This means a doctor must be informed as soon as the child has come into contact with the virus. Gammaglobulin comes from human blood and contains anti-bodies. It is used only in exceptional cases where a child has not been vaccinated but would suffer severely from contracting measles. For example this may occur if the child is already ill and weak. Gammaglobulin is only effective for two weeks.
Treatment and quarantine Measles is spread by tiny droplets from the nose and throat of an infected person. It is highly contagious from the day the cold symptoms first appear.

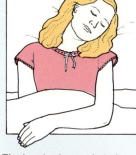

The incubation period, the time lapse between contracting the disease and showing the symptoms, is up to two weeks. Measles is so contagious that it would probably not restrict the spread of infection if the child were to be placed in quarantine within the home.

If a case of measles is suspected inform the doctor. There is no specific form of treatment except to keep the child comfortable. Paracetemol or soluble aspirin can be used if he has a high fever and a linctus may help relieve a bad cough. The child will probably want to stay in bed and is likely to be off his food, but this is no cause for concern. However, do ensure that he gets plenty of fluid.

The rash is not itchy and requires no treatment, but if the eyes are severely afflicted wash them gently with warm water. It is not usually necessary to keep the child in a darkened room.
Complications Measles can be uncomfortable for a child, but it is unusual for it to lead to further illness. In fact the only after-effect is life-long immunity to the infection. However, if a child is ill when he contracts measles, or if he is exposed to other infections while suffering from measles, there can be complications and secondary infections. These usually affect the throat, chest or ears. An extremely rare complication is encephilitas (inflammation of the brain).

If a high temperature persists beyond the normal period, or if the child fails to improve after the rash has faded, consult a doctor.

German measles (rubella)

GERMAN MEASLES IS CAUSED by the rubella virus, and in childhood it is a minor illness, with mild symptoms. However the rubella virus is so serious if caught by a pregnant woman that all girls should be immunized against it during their early teens before they start their reproductive period, even if they believe they have had German measles. Once a girl has had German measles she will not catch it again, but a problem with the disease is that it is difficult to diagnose. The rash is mild and variable and doctors can never be absolutely certain a child has had it so no girls should assume they are immune. Children known or thought to have rubella should not be allowed to make contact with women who are pregnant. They may remain infectious for up to a week after the start of the illness.

The incubation period for German measles is two to three weeks. It starts with a runny nose, and the glands in the neck become enlarged. The rash appears after a day or two, starting on the face and spreading down to cover the trunk and limbs over the next 24 hours. The rash, consisting of small flat red spots, fades rapidly from the face, and has usually disappeared altogether in about two days.

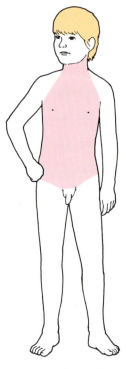

The rash The illustration above shows the sites of the rash. A typical rubella rash (see photograph) starts behind the ears and on the forehead and then spreads over the trunk. The tiny, flat pink spots are not itchy and may disappear in a day or two. The disease may be infectious from five days before until four days after the rash appears.

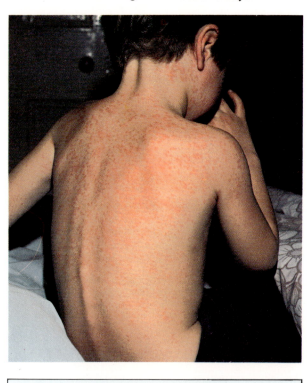

Congenital rubella

When a woman catches German measles in early pregnancy the embryo can become infected and this leads to abnormal development of the foetus, known as the rubella syndrome. Affected babies could be born with deafness, visual impairment, congenital heart disease, or mental handicap. They are usually of low birth weight, and there may be stunted growth. Children with the rubella syndrome continue to carry the virus for some years after birth, and can transmit infection to others. If a woman suspects she has German measles in early pregnancy she should consult her doctor. A blood test can show whether or not she has been infected, and termination of the pregnancy can be considered.

Summary

1. German measles is a mild infectious disease which does not usually cause children much discomfort. Complications are rare.

2. The danger is in infecting the unborn child, so it is essential for children to be isolated during the illness, particularly from pregnant women.

3. The incubation period is two to three weeks (see also immunization chart, page 48).

4. It is a difficult disease to diagnose because symptoms are mild and often the rash has disappeared before the doctor has seen the child. Consult your doctor if you suspect that your child has German measles.

Chicken pox

CHICKEN POX, ALSO KNOWN as varicella, is a viral illness characterized by crops of itchy pink pimples. It is highly contagious and attacks usually occur in childhood. One attack gives a child immunity to the disease. However, after the illness the virus may not be completely eliminated from the body, and can lie dormant for many years. Shingles (herpes zoster) is a local flare up of infection arising from this dormant virus. It mainly occurs in adults. Children can catch chicken pox from adults who have shingles as well as from contact with children with chicken pox.

The incubation period for chicken pox is usually between 13 and 17 days, but may vary slightly. The first day of illness consists of slight fever and discomfort, and within 24 hours the typical rash starts to develop. It starts as small raised red spots which very quickly become small blisters and are intensely itchy. After a day or so the fluid in the spots becomes cloudy, a scab forms and the sore gradually heals.

Over the first three or four days successive crops of spots erupt so the rash becomes more severe and extensive. The rash will consist of spots at various stages with red spots, small blisters, pimples and scabs at the height of the illness. The rash starts on the trunk, which remains the main site, but spots occur on the face and scalp, and to a lesser extent on the limbs. In severe chicken pox the spots develop on mucous membranes inside the mouth, and in girls the area around the vulva may be affected.

While the rash is erupting the child is ill with a fever, has a poor appetite, and is distressed by the itching. There is no specific treatment for chicken pox but the child should be discouraged from scratching, and a lotion, such as calamine, may soothe the itching. The doctor may give a mild sedative.

No new lesions appear after about four days, and existing lesions gradually heal. The child remains infectious until all the lesions have scabbed over or have disappeared, which is six or seven days from the start of the rash. In general, chicken pox does not leave permanent scars, unless any of the lesions become secondarily infected, usually as a result of scratching.

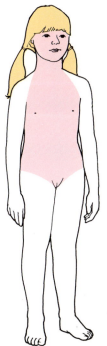

The rash The sites of the rash are indicated in the illustration above. The spots first show up on the body, face and in the scalp. Over the next few days more spots will appear on the trunk, in the armpits and groin, and they may extend around the eyes and in the mouth.

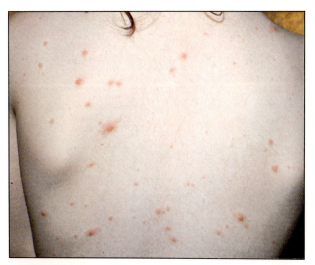

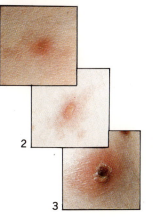

Spot formation The spots appear on the skin in crops over three or four days, until all three stages of development are present together (see above).
1. The first crop of spots is small and dark red.
2. In a few hours they fill with fluid and resemble blisters.
3. These dry into scabs and drop off, leaving a pink scar which soon fades.
The spots are very itchy and, if scratched excessively, will become infected so that antibiotic treatment may be necessary.

Summary

1. Chickenpox is a highly contagious disease.

2. The first signs of illness are fever and general discomfort, followed by the onset of a rash on the trunk and face.

3. The incubation period is two to three weeks.

4. Let your doctor know if you think your child is developing chickenpox.

5. When the scabs have formed, the child is no longer infectious.

Mumps

MUMPS IS A VIRAL disease characterized by tender swelling of the glands just in front and below the ears (the parotid salivary glands), but other parts of the body are often involved. Mumps is less contagious than measles or chicken pox and some children will escape infection throughout childhood. An attack of mumps gives permanent immunity.

The incubation period for mumps is 14 to 24 days. The illness usually starts with the development of pain and swelling of the parotid gland on one or both sides of the face. Within a few hours there is a pronounced swelling below the ear, which pushes the ear lobe upwards. The swelling extends forward over the lower jaw. If only one side of the neck is affected initially, the other side usually becomes infected within two days. There may also be swelling and pain in the glands under the jaw at the front of the neck.

The child will have a fever, even before the swelling, and will suffer pain and general discomfort from the swollen glands. The glandular swelling gradually subsides over four to eight days and the fever and pain settles over the same period. The patient ceases to be infectious when the swelling has gone down.

In most cases there are no other features of mumps infection, but sometimes other parts of the body are affected. The most usual complication is when the brain and its surrounding membranes are affected. This is know as mumps meningitis, or mumps meningo-encephalitis, and may occur before or after the neck swelling. A severe headache develops rapidly and the child will dislike bright lights, noise and movement. The temperature rises and vomiting may occur. If the child is known to have mumps the diagnosis is straightforward, but if there is no parotid gland swelling the child must be examined for other forms of meningitis. The doctor may need to perform a lumbar puncture to withdraw some of the cerebro-spinal fluid and establish the diagnosis.

If an adolescent or adult male develops mumps it can involve the testicles. It is rare for this to occur before puberty. Local swelling and pain of one, or both, testicles can start up to a week after the mumps has begun, and lasts for three or four days. This complication is called orchitis. It is accompanied by fever, abdominal pain, and nausea. When the swelling has subsided the testicle may appear softer and slightly smaller than before the illness, but infertility following mumps orchitis is very uncommon.

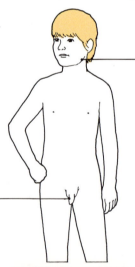

Symptoms A swollen and tender parotid gland is usually the first sign . One side often swells up a day or two before the other. The child will experience pain from the swollen glands and have a fever.

Orchitis This is a complication which occurs in adolescent boys and men. A week or two after swelling in the face, pain and swelling in one or both of the testicles can occur. These symptoms are accompanied by a high temperature, abdominal pain and nausea.

The illustration (right) shows a child with mumps. The left-sided parotid and submandibular glands are swollen. As well as the glands being enlarged, they are painful and tender to touch. The parotid gland (far right) is in front and below the ear (A). When it swells it pushes the ear lobe upwards. The submandibular gland (B) is under the jaw below the back teeth.

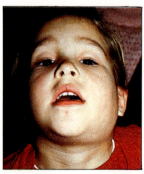

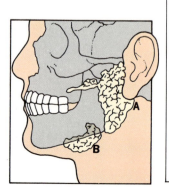

Summary

1. Mumps is not highly contagious, therefore some children will escape infection throughout childhood.

2. The incubation period is about three weeks.

3. A painful swelling of the neck (parotid) glands on one or both sides of the face is usually the first sign of mumps.

4. This is normally a mild illness but there are various possible complications such as mumps meningitis and inflammation of the testicles in adolescent boys and men.

5. The child is no longer infectious once the swelling has gone down completely. An attack of mumps gives total immunity.

Glandular fever

GLANDULAR FEVER (infectious mononucleosis) is an infectious illness which most commonly affects adolescents and young adults, but can occur at any age in childhood. The incubation period is about 10 days. Those who catch it have seldom had direct contact with anyone else who has the disease and, as features of the infection can be very variable, diagnosis may be difficult.

Fever is the most common symptom, coming on gradually or starting suddenly, and persisting for several days, or even a week or two. The temperature may go as high as 103°F (40°C) in the evenings but is usually normal in the mornings. The fever is accompanied by discomfort, lethargy and poor appetite. Many patients have a sore throat and headache, and occasionally there is a skin rash.

The virus of glandular fever particularly affects lymphoid tissue and when the doctor examines the child, he may find enlarged lymph nodes in the front of the neck, under the arms, and in the groin. The tonsils are usually enlarged, as is the spleen.

To confirm the diagnosis a blood count and a special glandular fever blood test is necessary. The blood contains an excess of mononuclear white blood cells in glandular fever, hence the alternative name, infectious mononucleosis.

There is no specific treatment for glandular fever. As the infection is due to a virus, antibiotics are of no benefit. General nursing care and temperature control with soluble aspirin or paracetamol is all the treatment available. Glandular fever can be prolonged and even when the fever has settled, the patient will be weak and lethargic for many weeks. It is unusual for glandular fever to be passed on by direct contact so strict isolation is not necessary.

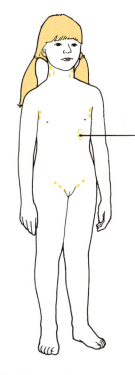

Enlarged Spleen The spleen often becomes enlarged in glandular fever.

The diagram above illustrates the main areas of lymph glands. In glandular fever the lymph glands of the neck, armpits and groin swell very obviously.

The equipment (see right) used in a blood count. A blood count is a test in which the number of red and white blood cells in a fixed volume of blood are counted. If a child has glandular fever the count will show the presence of an abnormally large number of white blood cells. The insert illustrates the virus known as Epstein Barr which causes glandular fever. The virus can lie dormant for up to seven weeks before it begins to multiply and attack the lymph glands.

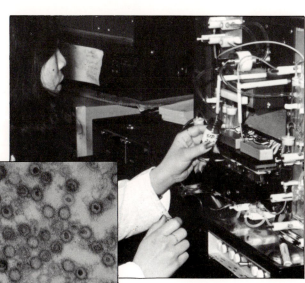

Summary

1. Glandular fever is an infectious illness which commonly affects adolescents and young adults.

2. Because it is not highly infectious strict isolation is not necessary.

3. The symptoms of glandular fever are fever, lethargy, headache, poor appetite and a sore throat.

4. There is no specific treatment for glandular fever and it can often last for many weeks.

Whooping cough

WHOOPING COUGH IS a highly infectious disease, which can affect people of all ages but is most serious in babies and small children. It is due to infection by a bacteria known as bordatella pertussis, and has an incubation period of one to two weeks.

The first symptoms are usually coughing and a runny nose, often indistinguishable from any other upper respiratory infection such as a cold or flu. This is the stage at which the child is most infectious, and it lasts for about a week. Gradually the cough becomes more severe and it is at this stage that whooping cough may first be suspected. The cough occurs in spasms with the child going red or blue in the face, being very distressed, and at the end of the spasm, vomiting a sticky mucus. After the spasm, breathing is noisy — the so-called 'whoop'.

Attacks vary in severity and not all children make a whooping noise. Coughing tends to be worse at night. There is gradual improvement but bursts of coughing, accompanied by choking and vomiting, may persist for two or three months. Even when whooping cough appears to be getting better, symptoms may become worse again if the child gets a secondary infection such

as a cold. These relapses may go on for up to a year.

A doctor will normally be able to diagnose whooping cough once the symptoms have become severe — after a gradual onset of coughing, becoming spasmodic and accompanied by vomiting, redness in the face and the 'whoop' in the child's breathing. Unfortunately it is less easy to diagnose in the early stages of the infection but, if it is suspected that a child has whooping cough the doctor may take a sample from the back of his throat by making him cough on to a sterile dish, or a blood test may be done. Even if these tests do not show up the infection there is still a possibility that the child has whooping cough.

There is no special treatment for whooping cough, and antibiotics have no influence once the symptoms have appeared, but they may be given to those who have come into contact with someone already infected. Cough medicine is usually tried to alleviate the cough, but it seldom gives much relief. Treatment is therefore restricted to good nursing, providing comfort and nourishment. In small children the severity of the disease may make it necessary for the child to be cared for in hospital.

Why it happens Whooping cough is a specific bacterial infection of the air passages — nose, throat, trachea, and bronchi. Although it starts like a cold with runny nose and slight cough, the mucus produced in the air passages becomes thicker and more viscous than usual as the result of the infection.

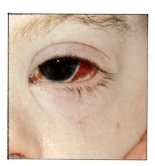

With the violent coughing in pertussis there may be conjunctival haemorrhage due to rupture of small blood vessels.

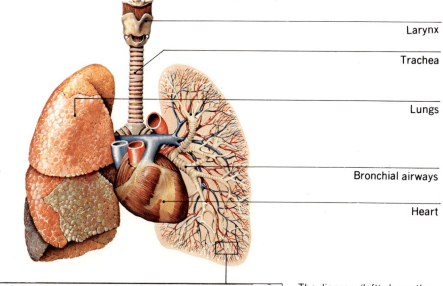

Larynx

Trachea

Lungs

Bronchial airways

Heart

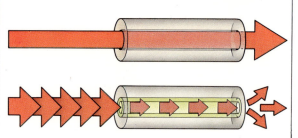

The diagram (left) shows the unrestricted path of air flowing through the bronchioles. When there is infection the airway becomes blocked with thick mucus so that paroxysms of violent coughing occur in order to dislodge the mucus and clear the airway (bottom left). After a bout of coughing the child may vomit thick mucus.

Home nursing of whooping cough

At first whooping cough is very similar to a cold with runny nose and slight fever. A cough develops, and when it has built up to a severe, repetitive paroxysmal cough the child can be quite ill and distressed. In severe cases hospitalization may be necessary.

No medication is effective in relieving whooping cough, so home nursing consists of general care of the child with attention to providing drinks and attractive meals and ensuring plenty of rest.

When the child has a coughing bout he may become very frightened and be unable to get his breath. A parent close at hand is reassuring. At the end of the paroxysm thick sticky mucus may be coughed up or vomited and should be wiped away with tissues or handkerchiefs.

During a paroxysm the child needs comforting, and firm banging on the back may help in bringing up the sticky secretion.

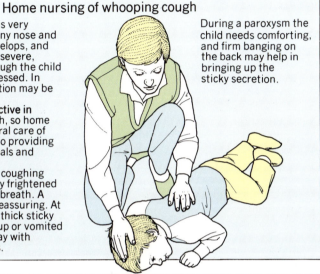

Summary

1. Whooping cough is a highly infectious disease, but it can be prevented by immunization.

2. Babies should be immunized against whooping cough at about three months old, six months and before they are a year old. This is part of the 'triple' vaccine, given with diphtheria and tetanus.

3. It starts with a runny nose and a slight cough.

4. It may take a week for the more serious symptoms to present. The cough gradually worsens, occurring in violent spasms with congestion of the face. Paroxysm may be followed by a whooping sound on inspiration, and by vomiting.

5. Symptoms can persist for three to four months. They are not greatly alleviated by any treatment, but sometimes cough mixture or antibiotics are given.

6. Whooping cough can be very serious, particularly for children under the age of two.

Reported cases of whooping cough

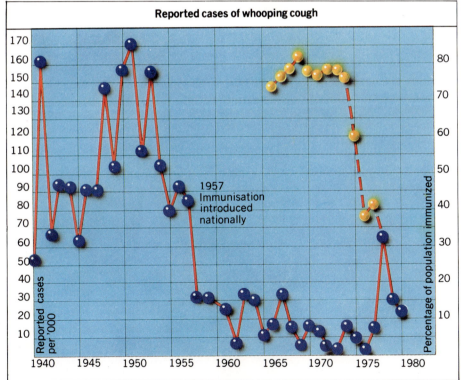

The relationship between immunization and reported cases of whooping cough is illustrated in the chart above which gives figures for England and Wales between 1940 and 1980. In the UK immunization was introduced nationally in 1957. Since then there was a steady decline in the number of reported cases of whooping cough until 1978 when there was a sudden increase. This increase was a direct result of the large fall in the immunization uptake rate. This fall was due to reports which suggested that the vaccine could cause brain damage. Since then a great deal of work has been done to find out whether the vaccine is really safe. It is generally agreed now that harmful side-effects from the vaccine are very rare indeed. As the vaccine is very effective the benefits of having the baby immunized far outweigh the risks of harmful side-effects.

Infectious hepatitis

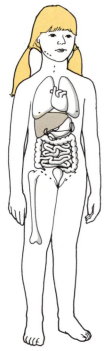

Infectious hepatitis is due to a virus which spreads through the body, but principally damages the liver There are symptoms of malaise, fever and jaundice.

THERE ARE TWO FORMS OF infectious hepatitis, known as hepatitis A and hepatitis B. The more severe kind is hepatitis B and it is rare in childhood. Infectious hepatitis A is seen occasionally in children, sometimes in small epidemics. It is very common in parts of the world with defective sanitation.

The incubation period is two to five weeks, and initial symptoms consist of poor appetite, fever, headache, nausea and vomiting. The child may complain of pain in the upper abdomen. After three or four days the jaundice appears. This is a yellowing of the whites of the eyes and of the skin. It varies in severity from slight discolouration only noted in the eyes, to a deep yellow pigmentation of the whole body.

With the appearance of the jaundice the fever usually subsides but weakness and loss of appetite persist while the jaundice lasts, and vomiting may continue. The time course of the illness is variable. Jaundice may last for only a day or two, or be prolonged for several weeks, but in most children improvement begins in about a week with increased appetite and gradual fading of the jaundice.

There is no specific treatment for infectious hepatitis. Affected children may infect others, and the virus is excreted in the stools during the illness. They should be isolated from other children if possible.

Injections of gamma globulin can often prevent the development of the disease if given soon after the initial contact, and should be considered for others in the family when one member develops hepatitis.

Summary

1. Infectious hepatitis A is sometimes seen in children. It occurs in small epidemics and is common in countries where sanitation is poor.

2. It is contagious.

3. The incubation period is two to five weeks.

4. The first signs of the illness are loss of appetite, fever, headache, nausea and vomiting. After three or four days the jaundice (yellow colouration of skin and eyes) appears.

5. There is no specific treatment for infectious hepatitis.

6. The length of illness varies. Generally in children improvement begins about a week after the jaundice has first appeared.

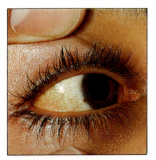

When jaundice presents there is a yellowing of the whites of the eyes (see above) and of the skin. Sometimes it is only the eyes that become slightly discoloured; at other times the whole skin takes on a deep yellow colour.

Prevention

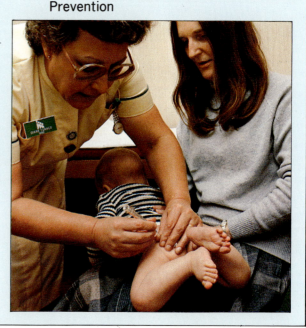

Infectious hepatitis is transmitted through the mouth by food and drink contaminated with the virus, and is excreted in the stools. If a child is infected the whole family must be very careful about hygiene, as the disease spreads most easily where hygiene is primitive. Hands should be washed thoroughly after using the lavatory and before meals. Injections of gamma globulin (right) can be given to individuals who are in close contact with infectious hepatitis to prevent the disease developing.

Tuberculosis

TUBERCULOSIS (TB) IS NOW uncommon in affluent societies, but infection may occur in children who have been in contact with someone who has the disease. All dairy herds are regularly tested, so milk is no longer a source of infection for children.

A child exposed to infection from TB develops a small infected lesion in the lung, and some reaction in the adjacent lymph nodes. The child may not appear significantly ill at this stage, and in many children the infection is overcome by the body's defences. Usually the local lesion heals and there is no further problem, but sometimes it does not heal and instead the infection spreads. This is particularly likely to happen to infants and young children, and in those who are undernourished. If the infection spreads locally the lung will become involved (pulmonary tuberculosis). If infection gets into the blood stream, it may spread around the body to other parts. TB meningitis, with infection around the brain, is the most serious manifestation of tuberculosis infection, but infection can occur in the bones, kidneys and other organs.

A child who has become infected with tuberculosis (or has been given BCG immunization), will show a positive tuberculin skin test reaction. This is a very important diagnostic test, but does not indicate whether or not the disease is active. This can only be done by Xrays, blood tests and attempts to identify the bacteria in sputum or stomach washings.

Tuberculosis responds well to treatment with appropriate antibiotics, but therapy needs to be continued for several months. Young children found to have a positive skin test are often given a course of treatment even if there is no other indication of active disease. This prevents the development of serious manifestations.

Immunization with BCG offers some protection against infection. BCG is a strain of live tuberculous bacteria which do not cause disease, but do activate the body defences against TB. It should be given soon after birth to children in communities where TB is common (among some immigrant groups and in socially disadvantaged areas). It should also be given to children in a family where another member is found to have TB. For other children it is given around the age of 13. BCG immunization is often provided at school.

Testing for past infection
About six weeks after infection with TB (or after BCG vaccination, which consists of an innoculation of a live non-pathogenic strain of TB) there is a change in skin reactivity. Injection of a bacterial extract into the skin (see right) produces no reaction in people who have not had tuberculous infection or a BCG, but provokes an inflammatory skin reaction in those who have (see inset). It does not indicate how recent the infection was, nor whether it is active. People who are skin test positive are less likely to get generalized infection if they again develop tuberculous infection.

There are various forms of skin testing, including the Mantoux test, Heaf test, patch tests, and tine tests. All work on the same principle.

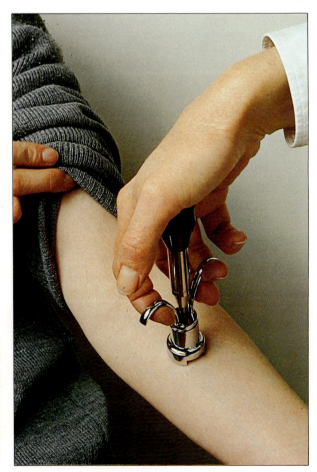

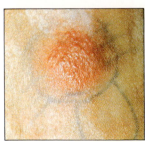

Summary

1. TB is no longer common in affluent societies.

2. When it does occur many children recover spontaneously, often without anyone realizing they had become infected.

3. In small children the infection can spread and cause serious disease.

4. Modern drug treatment is very effective against the infection, but treatment needs to be prolonged.

5. BCG immunization offers some protection.
See chart on page 49.

The Ear

STRUCTURALLY THE EAR CAN be divided into three parts, the external, middle and inner ears. The external is the part of the ear seen from the outside and is comprised of the pinna and lobe, which act like a funnel to receive the sound and direct it into the ear canal. The canal leads down to the ear-drum, or tympanic membrane, a thin taut layer of skin (like a minute drum skin) which vibrates whenever sound waves enter the ear.

The ear-drum divides the external from the middle ear. The middle ear is an air-filled space inside thick protective bone. Attached to the inner side of the drum is a chain of three minute bones, or ossicles, which move whenever the drum vibrates and transmit the sound from the drum across the middle ear to the inner ear. The cavity of the middle ear is connected to the back of the nose by the eustachian tube, and may predispose to infection. The middle ear also connects up with air spaces in the mastoid bone just behind the ear.

The inner ear consists of the organ of hearing, the cochlea, and the organ of balance, the semi-circular canals. The cochlea is a spiral tube filled with fluid and richly endowed with nerve impulses. The hearing

Balance

The inner ear contains an organ called the labyrinth which is made up of three semi-circular canals and the vestibule. Balance is regulated by the fluid in the canals, which are positioned at right angles to each other on either side of the head (see diagram below). The three canals are also at right angles to one another, one of them being horizontal (yellow), one vertical (blue) and one tilted (red). The end of the canals open into the vestibule and from here impulses are sent to the brain, providing information on the position of the head.

Structure of the ear The ear has three parts: external, middle and inner. The external ear is made up of the pinna and lobe. These act as a funnel to receive sound and then direct it into the ear passage. This passage, or external ear canal, leads down to the ear-drum which is a thin, taut layer of skin, also called the tympanic membrane. Beyond this is the middle ear, a small air-filled space inside thick protective bone. This cavity is bridged by three connecting bones: the hammer, the anvil and the stirrup.

The middle ear is linked to the back of the nose by the eustachian tube. This channels air from the nose to the middle ear in order to equalize the air pressure inside and outside the ear-drum. Without this, the ear-drum would rupture with sudden changes of pressure. Often, with a cold or hay fever, the ear will 'pop'. This is caused by a blockage in the eustachian tube clearing.

The inner ear contains the organ of hearing, the cochlea, and the organ of balance, the labyrinth. The cochlea is a spiral tube filled with fluid and containing many nerve endings. The labyrinth consists of three semi-circular tubes called canals.

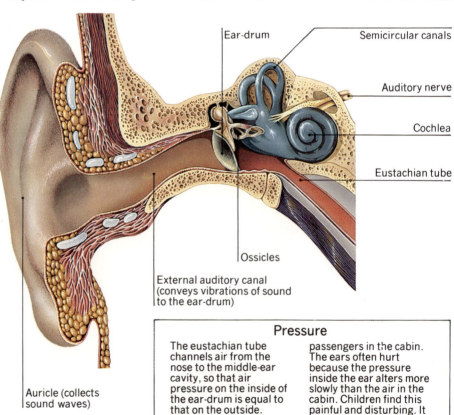

Ear-drum

Semicircular canals

Auditory nerve

Cochlea

Eustachian tube

Ossicles

External auditory canal (conveys vibrations of sound to the ear-drum)

Auricle (collects sound waves)

Pressure

The eustachian tube channels air from the nose to the middle-ear cavity, so that air pressure on the inside of the ear-drum is equal to that on the outside. Aircraft are pressurized, but when a plane is coming in to land the drop in height will affect the passengers in the cabin. The ears often hurt because the pressure inside the ear alters more slowly than the air in the cabin. Children find this painful and disturbing. It can be relieved by holding the child's nose while persuading him to try and blow out through it.

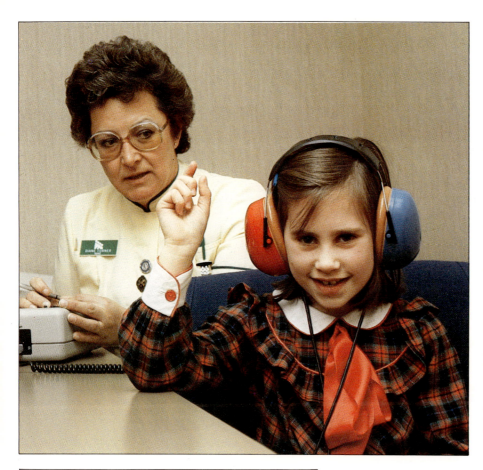

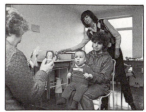

Hearing tests Regular hearing check-ups are a vital part of a child's medical routine from babyhood onwards. The first test is done at about six months old with the baby sitting on the mother's lap, looking forward. The tester makes a soft sound with a rattle or cup and spoon, on either side of the baby's head, out of visual range. If there is a definite response to these soft sounds the doctor can be confident that there is no major hearing loss. If the baby does not respond he is tested again and, if the results are still negative, referred to a specialist. Tests for pre-school children centre on games which require the child to respond to certain sounds. Older children are normally tested with a special instrument called an audiometer (shown left).

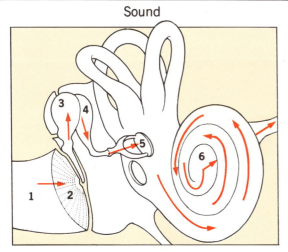

Sound

The external ear acts as a funnel for sound, directing sound waves down the external ear canal (1). When they reach the ear-drum membrane (2) the sound waves cause it to vibrate. These vibrations are transmitted and amplified from here through the middle ear by means of three bones: the hammer (malleus 3), the anvil (incus 4) and the stirrup (stapes 5). The vibrations then enter the cochlea (6), the central organ of hearing. The cochlea is a spiral containing fluid and thousands of cells covered in delicate hairs. These minute hairs move according to the sound they are receiving. They are tuned to vibrate to different sound frequencies. The hair-covered cells are surrounded by nerve endings which carry signals to the brain through the auditory nerve.

pathway is completed by the auditory nerve which carries input to the brain.

The semi-circular canals are also fluid-filled tubes embedded in bone. Movements of the head cause movement of the contained fluid, and the nerve endings convert this movement into nerve signals, which thus convey information concerning balance to the brain.

The development of hearing

Babies can hear and respond to sound by the time they are born. The spoken voice may be enough to settle the baby if he is awake and restless. Loud noises will startle the baby, who may respond by reflex, stretching out the arms and hands and crying. A newborn baby is not good at localizing sounds, but as head movements develop over the first few weeks, he will turn towards the source of sound with increasing accuracy.

As the baby develops he will start to talk back when he hears a voice, and this response provides the basis for speech development. Early vocalizations are mainly vowel sounds — oohs and aahs; by about six months consonants appear in the babble, and from this age the baby may try to imitate sounds. Impairment of hearing interferes with the development of communication and language, so it is important to detect any problem early.

Regardless of age, if you think your child is not hearing properly, you should seek expert advice, and your doctor will be able to refer your child to a specialist if necessary. Babies may respond to a parent's voice and still have a partial hearing deficit, so hearing tests are part of developmental testing for all children.

Ear infections

IN EXAMINING THE EAR the doctor inspects the outer ear, and looks into the ear canal with an auriscope (or otoscope) to see the canal and eardrum (tympanic membrane). The auriscope has a magnifying lens and a light source, and is inserted into the ear canal so that the doctor gets a magnified view of the canal and tympanic membrane. He will be able to see if there is excess wax, and whether there is infection or any other evidence of middle ear disease.

The doctor will also want to examine the nose and throat as they are closely related to the ear. He or she will feel the neck to see if there are any enlarged glands as this is often a feature of ear infection. The examination may also include a test of hearing using a tuning fork or other sound source. If there is any evidence of impaired hearing further hearing tests may be done.

Infection of the middle ear

The middle ear is connected to the back of the nose by the eustachian tube, and easily becomes infected when a child has a cold or other upper respiratory tract infection. In some children the ears are affected every time they have a cold. When the middle ear is infected the lining membrane becomes thickened and produces a mucus secretion. Hearing is likely to be impaired and there may be pain in the ear. Otitis media is the name

doctors give to infection of the middle ear.

Otitis media may be due to viruses or to bacteria, with bacterial infections being the most severe. The symptoms are very variable. Although temporary partial hearing loss on the affected side is usual, children may not be aware of this and therefore do not complain about it. There may be discomfort in the ear, varying from a dull ache to severe pain. In infants, rubbing or pulling the ear may suggest that the ear is infected. The child is likely to be miserable and irritable if the infection is severe, and the temperature may be raised. The lymph glands in the neck are likely to be enlarged and may be visible as a swelling below the ear.

Bacterial otitis media can be complicated by perforation of the eardrum, causing a discharge of pus from the ear. This is rarely seen if bacterial infections are promptly treated by antibiotics. Even less common is extension of the infection into the mastoid bone behind the ear, with pain and swelling developing in this area.

After an attack of otitis media the ears will usually return to normal once the infection has settled down. Occasionally the membrane lining the middle ear goes on producing excess mucus so that the ear remains full of fluid with consequent hearing loss. This is usually referred to as 'glue ear' (see page 66).

When doctors examine children with suspected ear

Ear infections can be caused by several different conditions and may affect the ear canal, the ear-drum, the middle ear or the eustachian tube. In order to detect the cause of the infection, the doctor will make a thorough examination of the inner ear using a medical instrument called an auriscope, or otoscope.

The diagram (below right) shows a view of the ear-drum, seen through the auriscope. If the ear-dum is normal the area marked by the cross will reflect the light. If the ear-drum is inflamed, indicating infection, there will be no light reflection, just a deeper red colour. If there is any perforation of the ear-drum (shown in diagram) a hole will be seen through the auriscope.

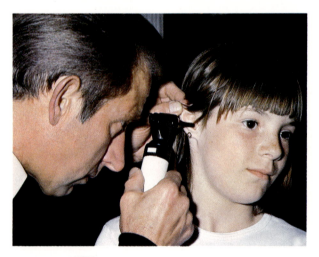

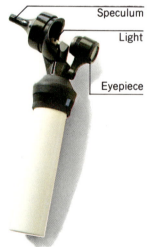

Speculum

Light

Eyepiece

The doctor will place the otoscope just inside the child's ear and look through the eyepiece. Light shines into the ear, showing up any abnormalities.

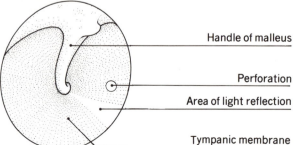

Handle of malleus

Perforation

Area of light reflection

Tympanic membrane

Wax blockage Wax is a natural secretion which cleanses the ear. When removing the wax from a child's ear, it is only necessary to wipe away any visible wax; never attempt to insert anything into the ear canal as you could cause serious damage.

It is not very common for children to get an accumulation of hard wax in the ear canal leading to a blockage, but this does sometimes occur. Symptoms can include earache, a ringing in the ears or even partial deafness.

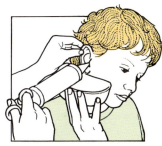

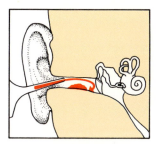

A blockage of wax in the outer ear-canal can be removed with a syringe containing warm water. The doctor will direct the syringe into the top of the ear canal and flush out the wax.

infections they may see a change in the appearance of the ear-drum. In acute otitis media the ear-drum is reddened and dull instead of its usual grey, shiny appearance. A throat swab may be taken in order to identify which micro-organism is causing an infection. If a bacterial ear infection is suspected, the doctor will start the child on an antibiotic, and usually the otitis media will settle over the next three or four days, resulting in relief of any pain and return of normal hearing. If there is perforation of the eardrum this usually heals spontaneously, but the doctor will need to check to make sure. Large perforations, which do not heal on their own, will need to be closed with a skin graft.

Infection of the outer ear

The ear passage of the outer ear is lined with special skin which produces the ear wax. This skin can easily become infected, or affected by skin diseases, such as seborrhoea — sometimes both happen together. The ear feels blocked and sore, the skin of the ear passage is red and thickened, and there may be a discharge of pus or a watery fluid. This is known as otitis externa.

Otitis externa can be treated with ear drops. If the condition is an infection, antibiotic drops are used, but if skin sensitivity seems the main problem, anti-inflammatory or combination drops are used.

Treatment of ear infections

Otitis media, or infection of the middle ear, requires treatment with appropriate antibiotics if it is thought to be due to a bacterial infection. Although the infection usually settles rapidly it may be followed by excess secretions into the middle ear — so-called 'glue ear'. This may also require appropriate treatment.

Otitis externa, or inflammation of the outer ear, may be due to bacterial infection, skin allergy, or other skin diseases. Treatment is usually with ear drops containing either an antibiotic, an anti-inflammatory agent, or both.

It is important not to damage the inner part of the ear when giving ear drops. Tilt the head to one side and squeeze the drops into the centre of the outer ear (1). Fold over the visible ear (2) and allow the drops to run inside.

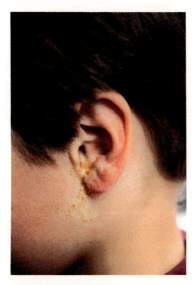

Otitis Externa Inflammation of the outer ear can cause deafness, pain and tenderness, and a copious discharge.

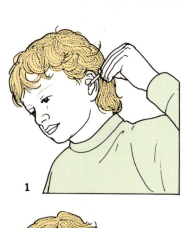

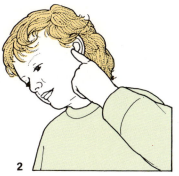

Loss of hearing

THE NORMAL EAR CAN hear very soft voices, a conversation in the middle of a crowded room full of people talking, and can pick up a wide range of sound, from deep bass voices to high pitched whistles. With a mild hearing loss it may only be the ability to hear the softest sounds that is lost, or an inability to hear high tones.

The child with a moderate hearing loss can usually hear well enough to learn speech and can take part in a conversation, but may find it difficult to concentrate on what is being said in a noisy room. A big handicap is that the child misses out on some learning opportunities by being unaware that a new event is happening, and also on a lot of casual communication with other people. The child with partial hearing may benefit from education in a special school where particular attention is paid to improving verbal communication.

When difficulty in hearing is due to a disease of the eardrum or middle ear, it is known as conductive deafness, as there is interference with the conduction of sound between the outside and the inner ear. Most acquired forms of hearing loss in childhood are of the conductive type, and there are various treatments available, depending on the cause.

Severe, or total hearing loss, is a very major handicap. If present from birth the child is going to have a great communication problem which will obviously affect relationships with other people. The child will experience great difficulty with language, and may not learn any useful speech. Alternative communication skills, including sign language and writing, have to be developed. A specialized teacher of the deaf should be involved as early as possible, and the child will have to attend a special school.

If hearing loss is due to disease of the inner ear, or the nerves of hearing, it is known as nerve deafness. Many forms of deafness present from birth (congenital deafness) are of the nerve deafness type. At present there is seldom any specific treatment available for nerve deafness.

Many children do not complain of a hearing loss as they do not realize that anything is wrong, and parents may not be aware that the child is hard of hearing. Instead the child may be thought of as inattentive or dull. Because of the hearing loss the child understands less of what is going on around him, and as a consequence may be easily distracted and develop difficult behaviour. If there is any doubt that a child is hearing correctly a specialist opinion should be sought.

'Glue ear'

Partial hearing loss in childhood is most commonly due to the condition known as glue ear, in which the middle ear becomes filled with fluid instead of air. This fluid interferes with movement of the eardrum and ossicles, (the hammer, anvil and stirrup bones) and impairs sound conduction. A child suffering from glue ear may, or may not, notice a loss of hearing. He could also complain of a popping feeling or discomfort in his ear.

The eustachian tube, which connects the middle ear with the back of the nose, normally opens on swallowing and equalizes the air pressure between the middle ear and the outside. Blockage of the eustachian tube leads to a negative pressure developing in the middle ear cavity. this negative pressure draws fluid into the ear from the lining mucous membrane. At first thin and watery, the fluid gradually becomes more gelatinous.

When an infection causes a problem in the eustachian tube it will usually settle in three or four weeks. The fluid within the middle ear drains away or is reabsorbed and hearing returns to normal. Treatment with antibiotics for the infection, and decongestants to dry up the fluid, may speed up the return of normal hearing.

If glue ear is persistent, or recurs frequently, surgical treatment may be necessary. Under an anaesthetic a

Ear-drum | Ossicles

Fluid in ear | Infection spreads up eustachian tube

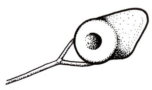

A grommet is a small plastic air tube which is inserted into the ear-drum to equalize the pressure on either side. It is left in place for some time and usually drops out of its own accord. If it does not, the doctor may remove it after a year to allow the ear-drum to heal.

Glue ear (above) is a common condition in childhood. The eustachian tube becomes obstructed, often by the adenoids at the back of the nose, so that air cannot get into the middle ear. The middle ear cavity fills up with fluid and the ear-drum is immobilized as a result. As time goes on the fluid becomes thicker and takes on the consistency of glue. If the condition is causing deafness, a myringotomy will be performed and a grommet inserted into the hole in the ear-drum for ventilation.

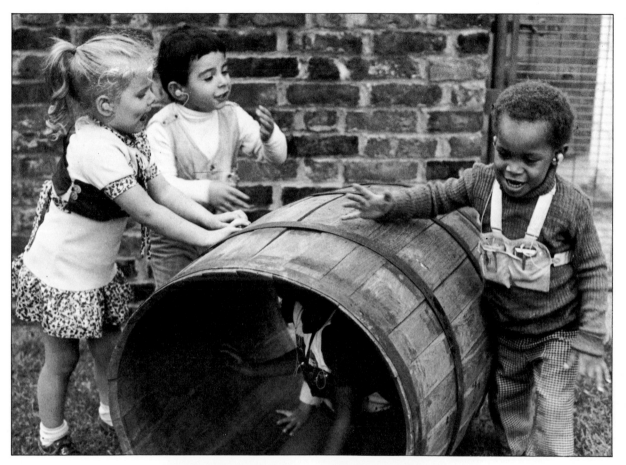

Hearing aids With young deaf children, one of the problems of wearing a hearing aid is keeping it securely in position and out of the child's way when playing or moving about. The hearing aid harness, worn by the children in the above photograph, is a stable unit which has either one or two pockets, depending on the number of aids required. It is comfortable and safe, and enables correct positioning for all body-worn aids.

The straps can be easily adjusted and the belt is fastened by a button and loop. Children can learn to put the harness on and off by themselves, which is important in school.

minute hole is made in the eardrum, an operation known as myringotomy. The fluid is drawn from the middle ear with a fine sucker. If the fluid is thick and jelly-like, a plastic tube called a grommet is inserted through the hole in the drum, and is left in place. This grommet acts as the eustachian tube and allows any remaining fluid to drain. It also prevents the development of negative air pressure in the middle ear.

When grommets are in place it is best not to allow water to enter the ear canal. Care is therefore necessary during hair-washing and swimming. A piece of cotton-wool smeared with vaseline should be inserted into the ears before starting either activity, and the immersion of the whole head in water should be avoided.

Grommets usually cause no discomfort. Occasionally the child may complain of popping, clicking or fullness of the ears. These mild symptoms settle quickly. However, if there is bleeding, discharge from the ear, or severe earache, the doctor should be consulted as soon as possible.

Grommets often fall out after a few months and the hole in the ear-drum heals over. Occasionally they may need to be removed when they are no longer needed. The adenoids are often removed at the same time as myringotomies are performed, if they are large and may be blocking the eustachian tube (see page 73).

Mouth and teeth

THE MOUTH COMPRISES the lips, cheeks, tongue and palate. The lips and tongue are highly mobile and are important in both talking and feeding. Furthermore, the mouth is a major tactile organ in babies as they put objects into the mouth to assess them.

The teeth usually start to come through at about six months, and the primary dentition (milk teeth), twenty in number, are usually all present by the age of two years. There is a marked variation in the timing of tooth eruption, but in most children the upper incisors, in the middle of the upper jaw, appear first. This primary dentition is gradually shed between the ages of five and twelve, with the replacement of larger permanent teeth thirty-two in number.

The mouth is kept moist by salivary glands. The largest of these glands are the parotids, situated just in front of the ear, one each side. They have a small duct which runs into the mouth on the inside of the cheek near the upper molar teeth. Two pairs of smaller salivary glands are situated under the tongue.

Mouth ulcers

Small painful ulcers of the mouth, called apthous ulcers, are common in some individuals. They come and go

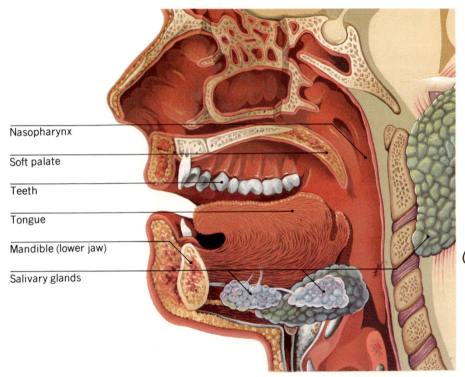

Nasopharynx

Soft palate

Teeth

Tongue

Mandible (lower jaw)

Salivary glands

The mouth consists of the palate, cheeks, teeth and gums, and tongue. At the back the mouth passes into the pharynx. The pharynx extends upwards to the back of the nose (nasopharynx), and downwards to the voicebox (larynx) and gullet (osesophagus).

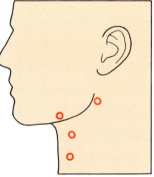

The lymph nodes in the front of the neck (shown above) may become sore and enlarged with infection in the mouth and throat.

The tongue consists of a complex system of muscles which make it extremely mobile. This enables it to deal with the functions of eating (swallowing and chewing) and speech. The tongue also bears organs that receive the sensation of taste. On the upper surface of the tongue there are minute hair-like projections called papillae which give it a velvety sheen. Within these papillae are numerous sensory organs (taste-buds). Four types of sensation are received from these taste-buds: salt, sweet, sour and bitter. Some areas of the tongue are more sensitive than others to particular tastes (right): sweet and salty are tasted at the front, sour at the edges and bitter at the back.

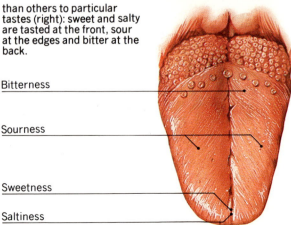

Bitterness

Sourness

Sweetness

Saltiness

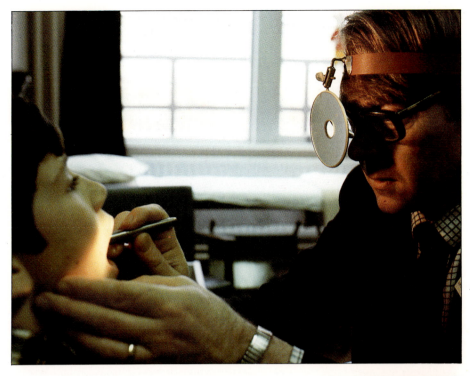

Examination of the mouth
The doctor looks into the mouth using light from a torch or head mirror (left). He looks at the tongue and teeth, and will look at the tonsils and back of the throat. A special mirror is required to see the adenoids. **Small painful ulcers** of the mouth are common (below left). Their cause is uncertain, but they may be helped by analgesic ointment or licorice extracts. **Thrush** (below) is a fungus infection which looks like milk curds. It is common in babies and after antibiotic treatment.
The detail below shows a microscopic view of candida albicans, the fungus which causes thrush.

over the space of a few days, but may be recurrent. They consist of shallow areas of about 0.5mm across, where the mucous membrane has disappeared, exposing the raw tissue underneath. The cause is unknown. Apthous ulcers need to be differentiated from ulceration which is caused by friction from a rough or broken tooth. Soothing applications prescribed by the doctor will give relief.

Thrush

Thrush consists of the appearance of white areas on the tongue and cheeks, due to a fungus infection called candida albicans. The lesions ressemble milk curds, but they cannot be wiped off.

Thrush is common in babies, who have little resistance to infection, and it can also occur in older children and adults, during or after an antibiotic course. Antibiotics can kill off the bacteria which normally inhabit the mouth, making it easy for the fungus to establish itself. There are several very effective antifungal remedies for thrush, including nystatin and amphotericin.

Dental Plaque and Caries

When a child eats a lot of sugary foods such as sweets, cakes and biscuits, particles of food remain on the teeth and encourage the growth of colonies of bacteria. These bacteria, known as dental plaque, remain firmly attached around the tooth gum margin and are difficult to remove by brushing. Plaque bacteria gradually erode the enamel on the outside of the tooth, and will then form a cavity in the tooth; this is known as dental caries. If unchecked, the tooth gradually decays and this may cause pain and discomfort for the child.

Children need to attend the dentist regularly from the age of three years and, if caries is detected in any tooth, a

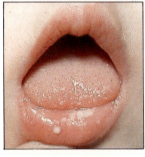

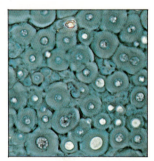

filling may be necessary. Prevention of caries is possible, with a threefold approach:
- Avoid sweets, biscuits and chocolates in the diet as much as possible.
- Brush the teeth thoroughly after meals.
- A small daily intake of fluoride during childhood will give teeth a resistance to caries. If the water supply is not fluoridated, fluoride tablets can be given. Alternatively, the teeth can be coated with fluoride by the dentist using a special process.

See also dental caries, page 29.

Enlarged glands in the neck

In some children enlarged glands (lymph nodes) are noted in the neck without any other indication of illness. They are usually a sign of septic illness around the mouth, throat or ears. The child should be carefully examined by the doctor and perhaps the dentist to see if a cause can be found. Treatment may be required.

Following an infection, enlarged neck glands may take months to subside to their normal size. When there are enlarged lymph nodes in the neck without any obvious cause, the doctor may want to do further tests. Tuberculosis and some other conditions can show up in this way.

The tonsils

THE TONSILS ARE SWELLINGS of lymphoid tissue present on each side of the throat, at the junction between the mouth and pharynx. Lymphoid tissue produces white blood cells and is part of the body's defence against infection. It grows rapidly in early childhood, and reaches a peak in size around the age of six or eight years, before gradually shrinking back in size during later childhood. This sequence can be seen in the tonsils: they are relatively small in infancy, prominent around the age of five, and have become noticeably smaller again by the age of ten. In some children the tonsils are so large that they appear to meet in the middle, but providing they are healthy, this is of no great importance, and they gradually shrink without treatment as the child grows.

Acute tonsillitis
The tonsils may become infected by bacteria or viruses giving rise to a sore throat. This may be part of a generalized upper respiratory tract infection associated with a runny nose and possibly a cough. If there is associated upper respiratory tract infection (URTI) the infection is probably viral and does not require specific treatment.

With bacterial infection, there is a sore throat, difficulty in swallowing, possibly a fever, and general malaise. The infection may well be localized to the pharynx and tonsils. The throat is bright red, and there may be some pus on the surface of the tonsils. The glands (lymph nodes) in the neck may be enlarged.

The doctor may want to take a swab from the throat to find out what is causing the trouble, and he will start treatment with an antibiotic to settle the infection. Usually there is significant improvement after about 24 hours.

Some children appear prone to recurrent attacks of tonsillitis. Provided the tonsils become normal between attacks, operative treatment is not usually necessary. Occasionally the doctor may recommend a prolonged course of antibiotics to prevent such attacks.

Tonsillectomy
The tonsils may become the focus of continuing infection after repeated attacks of tonsillitis. Sore throats are frequent and the child will probably have enlarged neck glands on one, or both sides. In this situation the doctor may recommend tonsillectomy, that is surgical removal of the tonsils.

Under an anaesthetic, the surgeon carefully cuts away the infected tonsils, and if the adenoids are enlarged, these may be removed at the same time. Following the operative treatment the throat is sore for a few days, but recovery is rapid.

Palate

Uvula

Inflamed tonsils

Tongue

The tonsils are situated on either side of the back of the throat. They consist of lymphoid tissue and form part of the body's immune defence system. It is normal for tonsils to be quite large in childhood. They reach their maximum size when the child is six or seven years old, and then gradually shrink. They also swell with infection, and may become chronically inflamed. A child who gets frequent sore throats and who has inflamed tonsils may benefit from their removal.

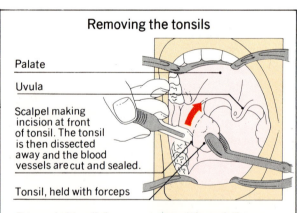

Removing the tonsils

Palate

Uvula

Scalpel making incision at front of tonsil. The tonsil is then dissected away and the blood vessels are cut and sealed.

Tonsil, held with forceps

Removal of tonsils is rarely indicated in children under the age of five years. If, however, the tonsils are the site of chronic or recurrent infection removal (tonsillectomy) may be indicated.

The child is anaesthetised and the head is extended backwards so that the surgeon can cut out the tonsils without danger of blood getting into the larynx (wind pipe). A tube passed through the nose into the larynx maintains the anaesthetic. The tonsils are dissected away from the wall of the throat, and all blood vessels are sealed to prevent bleeding. Recovery from the operation is usually rapid.

At the dentist

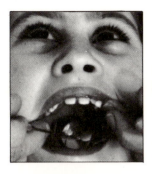

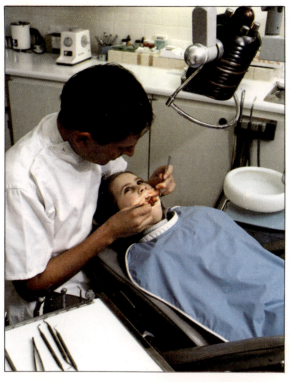

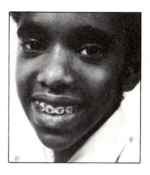

A child should visit the dentist regularly — about every six months. It is a good idea to take the child to the dentist before there is anything specifically wrong so that he gets used to the people and the place. His first visit should be at about three years.
What happens at the dentist At a check-up the dentist will examine the child's mouth for early signs of decay and the gums and mouth for signs of infection or other problems. He will use a mirror (see above) and a needle-shaped probe. Sometimes he may take an Xray to look for signs of decay which are not apparent on a visual inspection.
Milk Teeth It is important to look after them even though they are not permanent. Their premature loss can mean that the second teeth come through crooked and out of position. Cavities should be detected as soon as possible and a dentist's skill is needed to discover them when they are small. At an early stage it is far simpler to drill and fill them and it is unlikely to cause the child much distress.

Sometimes when permanent teeth come through, problems of overcrowded mouths and crooked teeth arise. Orthodontics is the treatment of crooked teeth and dentists usually start this treatment at about eight to ten years when most of the second teeth have emerged. Sometimes teeth are extracted in order to make room to move and straighten remaining ones. A brace (see above) straightens badly positioned teeth by placing a slow, continuous pressure on them. Some braces are fixed and stay in for months, others can be taken out and cleaned. Patience is needed as it is a lengthy, and sometimes uncomfortable process.

Formation of teeth

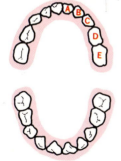

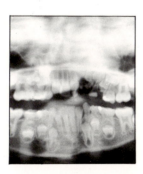

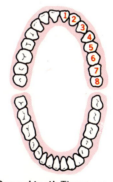

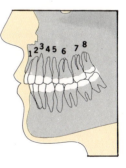

Milk teeth There are 20 milk teeth all formed under the gums before birth. The time at which they emerge varies widely from child to child.
The figures listed here are only averages. 1st and 2nd incisors: 6 - 13 months (a, b), 1st molars: 12 - 15 months (d), canines: 16 -18 months (c) and 2nd molars: 2 - 3 years (e).

Replacement of milk teeth The first permanent molars grow into place behind the milk teeth at about six years old; the milk teeth are then pushed out by their permanent successors. This is a painless process and there is virtually no bleeding at all.

Second teeth There are 32 teeth in a full adult set and these consist of four types: eight incisors (1, 2), four canines (3), eight premolars (4, 5) and 12 molars (6, 7, 8). The first permanent teeth to appear are usually big back teeth molars (6) at about six years old. The last set of teeth — the 3rd molars or wisdom teeth (8) can emerge as late as 25 years, if at all.

What they do Incisors are chisel-shaped and are used for biting off and cutting food.
Canines are tearing teeth.
Premolars work by a slicing action.
Molars are used for grinding food into small pieces.

The nose

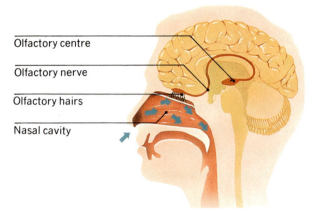

THE NOSE IS THE organ of smell and also has an important respiratory function in warming and humidifying the inhaled air. The nasal cavity has a large surface area, subdivided by thin bones covered with mucous membrane. This mucous membrane lining ensures that the air is warmed and moistened before it reaches the lungs so that they are protected from excessive variation in temperature, and from dryness. The pharynx is the muscular back-wall of the nose, mouth and throat. During swallowing the soft part of the palate contracts and closes off the nasopharynx to prevent food or fluid from getting into the nose. At the back of the nose, above the palate, are the adenoids. These are collections of lymphoid tissue which form part of the body's defence against infection. Sometimes the adenoids become enlarged and it may be necessary to remove them by an operation called an adenoidectomy. The eustachian tubes connect the middle ear to the wall of the pharynx on each side, near the adenoids.

Sense of smell Tiny particles, present in the air, are breathed in through the nose. They are transported to the nasal cavity where the olfactory hairs send impulses via the olfactory nerve to the olfactory centre of the brain. Here the various smells (fetid, fragrant, fruity, resinous and tarry) are distinguished.

Olfactory centre

Olfactory nerve

Olfactory hairs

Nasal cavity

The common cold
This is a virus infection familiar to all, consisting of one or two days of excessive watery discharge from the nose,

The nose is both the organ of smell and an organ of respiration. In normal breathing air is drawn in through the nose, where it becomes warm and moist before passing on to the trachea and lungs.

The olfactory organ, responsible for the sense of smell, is at the top of the nose and the nerve from it carries impulses to the brain.

The floor of the nose consists of the hard and soft palate. At the back the nose becomes the nasopharynx, connecting with the back of the mouth. The eustachian tubes from the ears enter the side of the nasopharynx.

Frontal sinus

Nasal cavity

Soft palate

Teeth

Nasopharynx

Tongue

Pharynx

Mandible (lower jaw)

Throat (larynx)

Oesophagus

followed by two or three days of thick muco-purulent discharge. Thereafter it usually clears up, but may predispose to cough, wheeze or ear infection in susceptible children.

There is no specific treatment; if the child is feverish, an ANTIPYRETIC such as paracetamol or soluble aspirin may help. In small babies who are still breast or bottle feeding, a cold can cause feeding difficulties as sucking from a nipple or teat requires breathing through the nose. In this situation decongestant nose drops, before the feed, may help.

Nose bleeds (Epistaxis)
The mucous membrane lining of the nose has a rich blood supply, and the nose bleeds readily if it is injured by a fall or a blow to the face. Spontaneous bleeding is also common in children who are otherwise healthy. The first aid treatment for nose bleeds is given on page 184.

If a child has recurrent nose bleeds it may be useful to have a specialist opinion. Some children can develop distended blood vessels on the nasal septum which rupture easily, either spontaneously or following nose blowing. The doctor may be able to shrink them by the application of cauterizing chemicals.

Foreign bodies in the nose
Small children may push small objects up their noses, and this will usually be realized by their parents at the time. To the inexperienced, the removal of such objects is difficult; attempts may only succeed in pushing the object further into the nose. They can usually be easily removed by the doctor with a specially designed hook.

Sometimes parents will not know that the child has anything stuck inside the nose, particularly if it is a soft object made of sponge or rubber. These can remain inside the nose and cause discharge or an offensive odour.

Enlarged adenoids
In early childhood the adenoids may become enlarged, causing nasal obstruction. The child becomes a mouth breather, and is likely to snore at night. Englarged adenoids also predispose to ear infections as they interfere with the function of the eustachian tubes. When enlarged adenoids give rise to significant symptoms their removal may be necessary; an operation known as adenoidectomy. Tonsillectomy (see page 70) is often performed at the same time. While the child is under an anaesthetic, the surgeon scrapes away the excess adenoidal tissue using a curved instrument inserted through the mouth. Adenoidectomy should restore the ability to breathe through the nose, and prevent recurrent attacks of otitis media, which is inflammation of the middle ear.

The adenoids are situated at the back of the nose, above and behind the soft palate. Like the tonsils they perform a useful function in protecting against infection in this area. Sometimes surgical removal is indicated if the child suffers from recurrent throat infections, earache or partial deafness, or the adenoids become enlarged causing nasal obstruction.

The adenoids can be examined by the doctor through a small mirror which is placed at the back of the throat and directed upwards. The adenoids are reflected in the mirror (right).

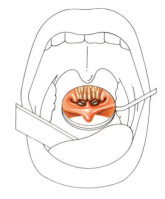

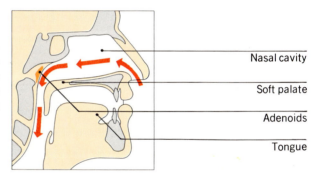

Nasal cavity

Soft palate

Adenoids

Tongue

Adenoidectomy

Enlarged adenoids obstruct breathing through the nose. The child becomes a mouth breather, and snores at night. Enlarged adenoids predispose to ear infections and glue ear, and may need to be removed.

Under an anaesthetic a special instrument is passed through the mouth up into the naso-pharynx, and the excess adenoidal material is scraped off. Tonsillectomy is often performed at the same time, and myringotomy (puncture of the ear-drum) may also be indicated.

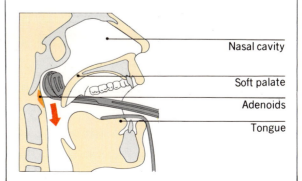

Nasal cavity

Soft palate

Adenoids

Tongue

Allergic disease and hay fever

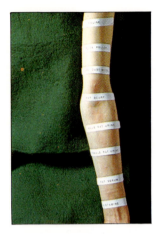

Hay fever In order to treat hay fever with desensitizing injections, the child will be required to undergo a series of skin tests (see above). The doctor will scratch a small spot on the child's arm and apply a few drops of liquid containing a common allergen. If the skin becomes red and itchy, the child is obviously allergic to that particular substance or substances which are causing the allergy and he can then start the relevant course of injections for treatment. Desensitization by injection is effective in about 75 per cent of cases.

AN ALLERGY IS AN untoward reaction of the body provoked by a particular substance (the allergen) which is usually a protein foreign to the body. Allergic reaction may be localized to one organ such as the nose, lungs, intestines, or skin, or may be generalized. Allergens may be particular foods, inhaled dusts, spores or pollens, substances which come in contact with the skin, or can be medicines or injections.

Certain individuals are particularly prone to develop allergies, perhaps on a basis of inherited predisposition or because of factors which may be aggravated by their emotional make-up, an important consideration in allergic disease. Allergic factors play a part in the development of the Atopic syndrome (which consists of *eczema, asthma* and *hay fever*) and atopic individuals readily develop other allergies. Some foods, such as shellfish and strawberries, induce allergies in many people.

Hay fever

Hay fever is a very common allergy of the nasal mucous membrane due to the inhalation of grass pollen. It is thus seasonal in early summer. Other pollens may provoke a similar reaction in which symptoms may be prolonged.

When pollen is inhaled by susceptible individuals the mucous membrane of the nose becomes swollen and congested, and produces a copious watery secretion. In a bad attack, the conjunctivae of the eyes may also be involved. Hay fever symptoms worsen on close contact with flowering grass, and when the weather is hot and dry so that the pollen count is high.

Hay fever sufferers are seldom able to entirely avoid contact with the allergen during the pollen season, so are likely to require specific treatment. A NTIHISTAMINE drugs taken orally can relieve the congestion and lessen the nasal secretions in many sufferers. Unfortunately in many people drowsiness is a side-effect (heightened by alcohol) and this limits the usefulness of the drugs in such cases. Antihistamine nasal drops and sprays may prevent any unpleasant side-effects.

Regular use of a preparation of sodium cromoglycate used locally as nasal drops or as an inhaler may prevent the onset of hay fever symptoms, and a locally active steroid preparation can benefit some people. Often, the particular irritant can be identified by sensitivity tests.

Desensitisation, using repeated injections of pollen extracts in an increasing dosage, can benefit some patients, but the injections may also provoke attacks in individuals who are very allergic to pollen.

Allergic rhinitis

Grass pollen is a seasonal nasal allergy. Some people have multiple nasal allergies, and may suffer from nasal

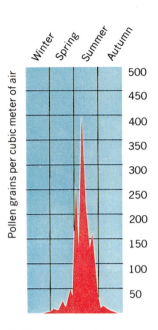

Pollen count Any airborne substance from a living organism can provoke an allergic reaction in a sensitive person, but the most common cause of hay fever is pollen. The pollen count is an index of the amount of pollen in the air at a particular time. It is highest in summer (see diagram above), and this is therefore the hay fever 'season'. Children who suffer from hay fever should be kept inside as much as possible when the pollen count is high. Details of the pollen count are usually given out by the media in the weather news.

congestion and excess secretion throughout the year. This is known as allergic rhinitis and treatment is along the same lines as that recommended for hay fever.

Food allergies

In sensitive individuals, an allergy to a particular food may provoke a reaction. This can take the form of intestinal disturbance, such as vomiting or diarrhoea, skin rash, or wheezing due to bronchospasm.

Babies with cow's milk protein allergy may experience vomiting, or failure to gain weight satisfactorily, with or without diarrhoea. Withdrawal of cow's milk from the diet may have a dramatic effect. Such dietary exclusion needs to be done under the supervision of a doctor or dietitian to make sure the baby's diet remains nutritionally adequate.

In severe *eczema* doctors sometimes think it is worth considering a trial of selective dietary exclusions to see if this will improve the skin.

Other allergies

Rashes, headaches, abdominal pains, over-activity and behavioural problems are sometimes blamed on food allergies. Undoubtedly in some children there may be allergies which manifest in this way, but unless a definite precipitating foodstuff has been identified, caution is needed in excluding too many foods from the diet. Eating a varied diet is a good protection against developing vitamin deficiencies and other nutritional problems.

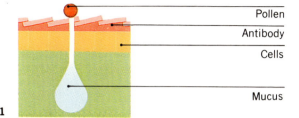

1 — Pollen / Antibody / Cells / Mucus

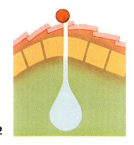

2

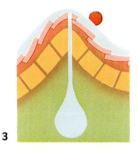

3

Pollen overkill The nasal lining of a hay fever sufferer contains antibodies which react to certain kinds of pollen. When pollen comes into contact with an antibody (1) an excess of fluid is produced, causing the tissue around the nasal lining to become swollen (2). As a defence mechanism, a large amount of mucus is secreted onto the surface of the nasal lining to attack and disperse the pollen (3).

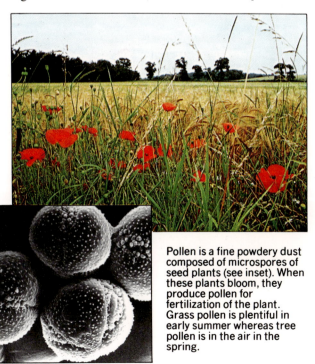

Pollen is a fine powdery dust composed of microspores of seed plants (see inset). When these plants bloom, they produce pollen for fertilization of the plant. Grass pollen is plentiful in early summer whereas tree pollen is in the air in the spring.

Allergy treatment

Some hayfever sufferers may benefit from a course of desensitization injections carried out in the preceding winter (see page 74). Nasal inhalation of sodium cromoglycate regularly during the pollen season will prevent the development of symptoms in some individuals. Nasal drops or spray of locally acting steroids may give marked benefit, as may steroid eye drops. Treatment with oral antihistamines may dry up the excess secretions, but can cause drowsiness.
Babies with cow's milk protein allergy may improve dramatically when cow's milk is withdrawn from their diet. This dietary exclusion must always be done under the supervision of a doctor to ensure that the baby's diet remains nutritionally adequate.
Common food allergies: strawberries, crab, shellfish and eggs can sometimes cause a reaction and should be excluded from a child's diet. Again this dietary exclusion must be done under the supervision of a doctor or dietitian.

The respiratory system

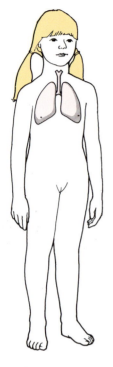

THE BODY CANNOT FUNCTION without air for more than a few minutes because it needs oxygen. The oxygen is present in the air and enters the bloodstream by way of the respiratory organs of the body. The respiratory system comprises the nose, throat, voice box (larynx), windpipe (trachea) and the lungs. Oxygen is needed in all parts of the body. It is carried by the blood to the tissues, where it is exchanged for carbon dioxide, which the blood carries to the lungs. This exchange of gases in the body is called internal respiration. The opposite exchange in the lungs, where oxygen is taken in and carbon dioxide breathed out, is called external respiration. The air passages leading to the lungs are kept moist by mucus, which helps to clear the air we breathe of any dust particles.

All the respiratory organs are susceptible to infection and there are many obvious symptoms which indicate respiratory disease:

Coughing is the mechanism for clearing the airways of any excess mucus, and an occasional cough is normal. Anything which irritates the airways, or which causes the production of excess mucus will induce coughing.

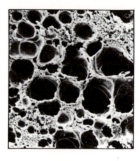

At the tip of each bronchiole is a minute balloon-like air pocket called an alveolus. There are millions of these alveoli in each lung and it is through the tiny blood vessels in the walls of the alveoli that the vital exchange of gases occurs. Because the wall of the alveolus is very thin, the blood capillaries which surround it are in close contact with the air. The alveoli extract oxygen from the air and remove carbon dioxide and water from the blood.

The lungs are the centre of the respiratory system. Air goes in and out of the lungs via the respiratory tract — the nose, throat and windpipe. Several muscles help to move air into the lungs, the principal of these being the diaphragm which lies between the chest cavity and the abdomen and is attached to the lower ribs. Between the ribs are the intercostal muscles which also help.

When the diaphragm contracts it lowers the pressure around the lungs and this causes them to expand, taking air into the respiratory tract. When the muscles relax, the lungs contract forcing air out.

Larynx (voicebox)

Right lung

Right main bronchus, air-tube of the lung, which divides into smaller bronchi and bronchioles

Aorta, main artery carrying oxygenated blood from the heart to the rest of the body

Trachea (windpipe)

Bronchioles, leading to alveolar duct

Pulmonary artery carrying blood to the lungs

Pulmonary veins return blood from the lungs to the heart

Bronchial airways

Heart

Exchange of gases in the alveolar sac

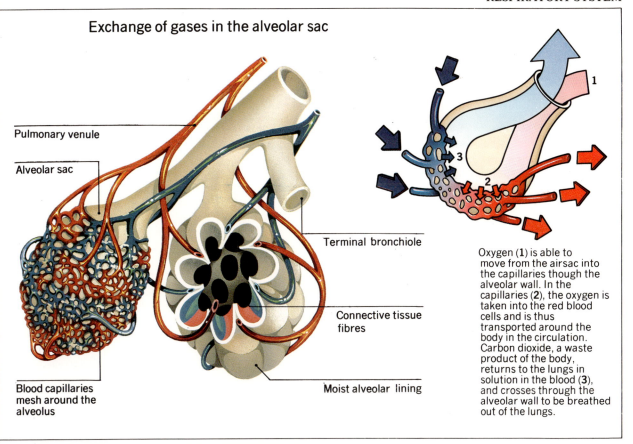

Pulmonary venule

Alveolar sac

Terminal bronchiole

Connective tissue fibres

Blood capillaries mesh around the alveolus

Moist alveolar lining

Oxygen (1) is able to move from the airsac into the capillaries though the alveolar wall. In the capillaries (2), the oxygen is taken into the red blood cells and is thus transported around the body in the circulation. Carbon dioxide, a waste product of the body, returns to the lungs in solution in the blood (3), and crosses through the alveolar wall to be breathed out of the lungs.

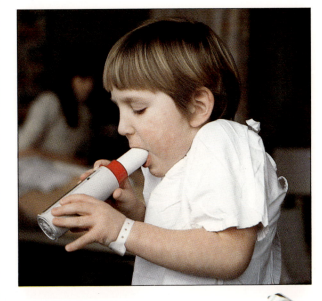

A peak flow meter is a small machine which measures breathing efficiency. It is used in the assessment of asthma and breathlessness.

The child is required to blow hard into the machine and, by measuring the maximum flow of air when breathing out, the doctor can assess the severity of an attack.

There are several other lung function tests, using more complicated apparatus.

Infection often causes an excess of fluid production and gives rise to coughing. This occurs with infection of the upper airways as well as with infection of the lungs themselves. Nasal secretions, as a result of a cold or hay fever, may be accompanied by a cough as some of the secretions will run down the back of the nose and collect in the throat. This is more likely to occur when the person is lying down, so a cough associated with upper respiratory infections tends to occur at night.

Noisy breathing is usually a result of some partial obstruction of the airways and children who snore at night may have some nasal obstruction. If this is persistent it may indicate enlargement of the adenoids (see page 73). Narrowing of the voicebox (larynx), often as a result of infection, gives rise to noisy breathing, loudest on breathing in. This is called stridor or croup, and is often accompanied by a hoarse voice and a cough which sounds like the barking of a seal (see page 82). Narrowing of the small airways gives rise to wheezing.

Wheezing is one of the most common symptoms in childhood. It consists of noisy breathing which sounds like whistling, and is usually accompanied by coughing and shortness of breath. It is due to a narrowing of the small air passages in the lungs and may be caused by asthma, bronchitis, or bronchiolitis.

Shortness of breath. Difficulty in breathing is always serious, and demands a medical opinion. It can occur in respiratory diseases in which there is narrowing of the air passages or infection of the lung. It can also occur with anaemia, and with some diseases of the heart and circulation.

Asthma

ASTHMA IS A WIDESPREAD and distressing complaint. During an attack, the small airways of the lung become narrowed and this causes wheezing and breathlessness.

There are many factors to be taken into account when looking for the cause of asthma and a great deal of research has been carried out in recent years. The main causes of asthma attacks include allergy, infection, strenuous exercise and emotion, but only if a child is susceptible to the disease.

Asthma is frequently associated with eczema and with hay fever, and if a baby has eczema in the first few weeks of life he may have asthma later in his childhood. The tendency to asthma is often hereditary so that if a parent or other close relative in the family has asthma or hay fever, a child is more likely to suffer from it also.

Attacks can be provoked by contact with a substance to which the child is allergic. Dust, grass pollens, and animal hairs are common allergies and it is worth trying to track down the allergy by recalling details about the period before an attack. Was the child in contact with a pet or other animal? Was the child playing in a dusty cupboard?

Attacks of asthma in young children are often set off by a cold or other infection, and a short while after the development of a runny nose the child may start to cough and wheeze. It may be thought that this is due to the infection spreading down to the chest, especially if the child is not known to be asthmatic. However, if this becomes a common occurence when the child has a cold it will become apparent that it is due to asthma.

Young children are common sufferers of asthma. It is unusual for a baby to have attacks in the first year, but it can start in the second year or at any time after that. However, it usually improves in later childhood and most children completely outgrow the tendency to wheeze in their early teens. In some children asthma

In susceptible individuals various stimuli alone, or in combination, may precipitate an attack. The items listed in the boxes do not cover everything and often it is not easy to isolate the cause of the problem. For example, a child might be excited about starting a new term at school, but he could also be wearing a woolly vest and both or either of these factors could cause an asthma attack.

Drugs A few drugs, particularly those called beta blockers, can worsen asthma in susceptible individuals. Beta blockers are only occasionally used in treatment for children.

Allergens Many asthmatic children have allergies to particular things. Very common are allergies to house dust, feathers, animal fur and grass pollens. Some children are also allergic to particular foods

Environmental Factors Pollution from fumes and other substances in the atmosphere can bring on an asthma attack. Equally they can be provoked by grass pollens. The most common factor in the environment to cause asthma is the house dust mite which is found in bedroom dust. Certain measures can be taken to reduce their numbers (see right), but they can never be completely eliminated.

Infection Colds and other upper respiratory tract infections often precipitate attacks of asthma in young children.

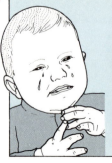

Emotional factors Attacks of asthma can be brought on or made worse by emotion. Crying, excitement or disappointment— whether pleasant or unpleasant — can provoke attacks.

Weather Rapid changes of temperature from hot to cold or from cold to hot can start an attack of bronchospasm. Some children are worse in damp weather; on the other hand children who are allergic to grass pollen may be more likely to get asthma attacks in dry weather in the spring.

Exercise Moderate or strenuous exercise will bring on an attack of wheezing in many asthmatic children. They may require treatment before undertaking sporting activities.

Controlling asthma in the home

House dust mites are one of the most common causes of asthma. They are so tiny that they can not be seen without a microscope and they live anywhere and everywhere in the house but prefer the bedroom most of all. The house dust mite is so ubiquitous that it is very difficult to eliminate entirely from a house; however certain steps can be taken to reduce the number of mites.

Things to do
1. The mattress, pillows and the base of the bed should be thoroughly vacuumed and the mattress should be enclosed in a plastic cover.
2. Quilts and duvets containing feathers should be exchanged for others which have a synthetic filling. The pillow should be filled with foam.
3. Every week the skirting boards, window sills and the plastic mattress cover should be damp-dusted. The pillow-cases and sheets should be changed and washed regularly.

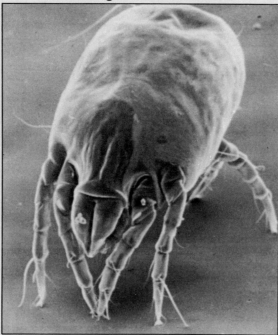

The house dust mite (above) can only be seen under a microscope. It lives on the scales of dead skin that human beings are shedding all the time, and is found especially in bedroom dust.

4. Blankets and bedroom curtains should be washed frequently.
5. During sunny periods the bedding should be aired as sunlight kills the mite.
6. If the child shares a bedroom, the same treatment must be applied to the other beds.
7. The child should be out of the room, and preferably out of the house, when the beds are made.
8. Other rooms should also be vacuumed carefully.

---

gradually gives way to hay fever and this is less troublesome than asthma.

Examination and prevention

For children who have infrequent attacks of mild asthma, diagnosis and treatment are usually straightforward and no special investigations are required. If the asthma is more severe the doctors may want to do special tests to assess the disease, including Xrays, lung function tests, and allergy testing.

Chest Xray. This is only of limited value in asthma, but in a severe or long and acute attack it may reveal an area of infection or lung collapse which was not detected by the doctor on physical examination.

Lung function tests. There are several tests which measure how the air gets into the lungs and out again. In the main they consist of breathing into machines which measure the air volume and flow rates. Lung function tests can be used both for diagnosis and for assessing progress. To assess the severity of the disease and response to treatment it is usually only necessary to measure how rapidly the patient can breathe out, by puffing into a machine called a peak flow meter.

Allergy testing. For selected patients it may be useful to do allergy tests. As some attacks are caused by the patient coming into contact with something to which he is allergic, a knowledge of the offending substance may help in prevention. Allergy tests are done by prick testing — injecting minute amounts of various materials under the skin to see if they cause a reaction. Allergy tests are occasionally done by making the child inhale the suspected substance. Positive reactions occur most commonly to house dust, the house dust mite (a microscopic insect found in house dust), pollen, feathers, and animal fur.

Attacks of asthma cause such distress to the child, that every step should be taken to prevent them. Attacks may be provoked by contact with feathers, animal fur, and dust. The replacement of feather pillows and quilts by cotton blankets and foam pillows may benefit many children. House dust is to be avoided, so the child should not be in the room during dusting or bedmaking, and preferably an hour should be allowed for the dust to settle before returning to the room.

Plastic or linoleum floorcovering in bedrooms causes less dust than carpets or wooden floorboards. A plastic mattress cover is also helpful in reducing dust.

It is unwise to get a furry pet for a child with asthma as the fur may start an attack. Guidance is more difficult if the family already has a pet. Removing the pet will sometimes have a markedly beneficial effect on the asthma, but not always, and there is often distress at the loss of a pet.

In spite of general precautions the child may continue to get frequent attacks, and the doctor may recommend the regular use of a drug called cromolyn sodium (Intal) which has to be breathed in through a special inhaler. The drug is less use during an attack, but it will decrease the severity of attacks in most asthmatic children if used regularly.

Physiotherapy may be part of the treatment for asthma and breathing exercises are taught to some children. They are aimed at teaching the child how best to use the lungs and reduce anxiety and discomfort during an attack. Physical exertion may provoke wheezing in susceptible children, but moderate exercise is to be encouraged. Swimming seems less likely to induce an attack than most other forms of exertion, and is an activity enjoyed by many asthmatic children.

Treatment of wheezing

Not all asthma attacks can be prevented, and when the child is having a bout of wheezing a drug which dilates the narrowed bronchial airway is needed. Bronchodilator drugs in common use for children include Albuterol, Terbutyline and Aminophylline and their derivatives. Bronchodilator drugs may be given as tablets or syrup, but act faster if inhaled. A supply of a bronchodilator should be kept handy for any child known to be liable to asthma since attacks occur without warning and often at night. If none of these measures seem to be helping in an attack, the child may become very distressed and exhausted and the doctor should be called. He may give an injection, or arrange admission to hospital.

Attacks can be alleviated by steroid drugs. The side-effects associated with the use of steroids are much reduced if the steroid is inhaled as an aerosol and this form may be prescribed if preventative measures and bronchodilator drugs are insufficient for control of the disease.

Special schools

Some children with asthma suffer considerable disability and may miss much of their schooling. For such children, asthma is a major handicap restricting both school and play, but improvement in adolescence is usual and an optimistic outlook should be maintained. Asthmatic children can be considered for entrance to open air schools.

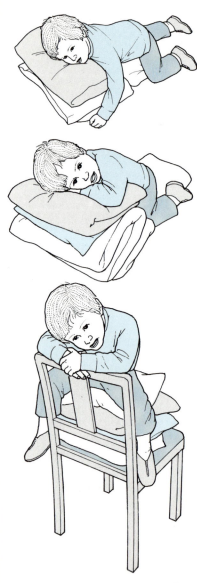

In an asthma attack the child needs to be positioned comfortably. He or she will be breathless, and may quickly become exhausted with the work of breathing. An upright, or semi-upright, position helps the breathing, and the illustrations above give a guide to some different ways the child can be nursed comfortably.

Children with asthma should as far as possible avoid things they know they are allergic to. In mild asthma, with only occasional attacks and with no wheezing in between, it is only necessary to use medication in the attack. With more severe asthma, with frequent attacks, or with some wheezing much of the time, drug treatment may need to be continuous, and the child will need frequent medical supervision. The doctor will want to know about the frequency and severity of the attacks, and will want to do occasional simple tests of lung function to assess the effect of treatment. Some d ugs for asthma are given as liquid medicine or tablets, but some are given into the lungs directly. There are various types of inhalers in use, including nebulizers driven by compressed air or an electric pump, pressurised aerosols, and inhalers which deliver the content of a capsule when the child breathes in.

Day		1	2	3	4	5	6	7
Number of Spincaps taken that day—		3	3	3	3	3	3	3
COUGH	None / Occasional / Often	0/1/2	0/1/2	0/1/2	0/1/2	0/1/2	0/1/2	0/1/2
WHEEZE	None / Occasional / Often	0/1/2	0/1/2	0/1/2	0/1/2	0/1/2	0/1/2	0/1/2
ENERGY	Usual self / Easily tired / Mostly inactive	0/1/2	0/1/2	0/1/2	0/1/2	0/1/2	0/1/2	0/1/2
PLAY/GAMES	Normal / Slight cough and/or wheeze / Severe cough and/or wheeze	0/1/2	0/1/2	0/1/2	0/1/2	0/1/2	0/1/2	0/1/2
MEALS	Usual self / Some interest / No interest	0/1/2	0/1/2	0/1/2	0/1/2	0/1/2	0/1/2	0/1/2
SLEEP	Normal / Mildly disturbed / Poor night	0/1/2	0/1/2	0/1/2	0/1/2	0/1/2	0/1/2	0/1/2
TOTAL SCORE		0	0	0	2	5	2	
REMARKS								

Asthma diary Keeping a full account of each attack of asthma may help to identify precipitating factors, and may help the doctor to plan treatment.

Treatment of asthma

Capsule inhalers (spinhalers)

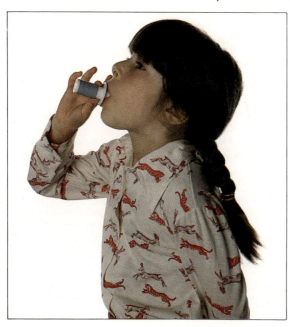

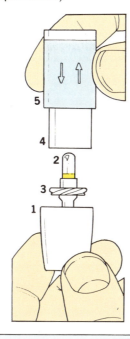

These inhalers can be used by children because they can be loaded quite easily and the drug capsule can be activated as required.

The diagram on the left shows an inhaler being loaded with a new capsule. With the mouthpiece (1) pointing downwards, the body of the inhaler is unscrewed and the drug capsule (2) is inserted into the centre of the propeller (3). The body (4) is then screwed back onto the mouth-piece and, by sliding the outer part of the inhaler down (5), the capsule will be pierced ready for use. The head must be tilted back and the mouth sealed over the mouth piece. When the child breathes in the propeller will be activated to release the drug.

Nebulizers

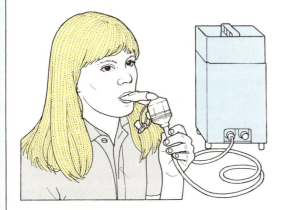

A nebulizer produces a shower of fine droplets that can be breathed in by blowing compressed air through a reservoir containing a solution of the bronchodilator drug. Younger children who may find it difficult to operate an aerosol (see right) manage best with a compressor nebulizer which delivers medicine through a face mask over several minutes. In hospitals, the compressed air or oxygen is used to nebulize drugs used in the emergency treatment of asthma.

Aerosols

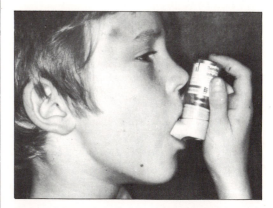

Pressurized aerosols are a convenient and effective way of giving small doses of broncho-dilator drugs directly into the lungs. The child should first breathe out and then seal the mouth around the mouthpiece (see above). It is important to coordinate pressing the aerosol with inhalation so that, as the child breathes in, a fine spray of the drug is inhaled into the lungs. Young children may find this difficult, so other treatment is best. Aerosols should not be used more than the prescribed amount.

Croup

CROUP IS ONE FORM of obstructed breathing caused by a narrowing of the larynx due to infection. Because of the narrowing breathing becomes difficult and noisy. The sound made is characteristic and is known as stridor or croup.

Croup most commonly occurs as a complication of a virus infection, and the term laryngo-tracheo-bronchitis is sometimes used to describe this infection which spreads down the air passages. It is unusual in children over the age of five years. Croup may be preceded by a day or two of the child feeling unwell and having a runny nose. The breathing difficulty starts suddenly, and usually at night.

The extent of breathing difficulty varies. For some children there will be only a slight increase in the rate of breathing, while more severely affected children will have to work hard to breathe and will be very distressed. There is often coughing and this too sounds croupy.

The way the illness develops is also very variable. There may be increasing difficulty in breathing as obstruction in the larynx gets worse; it may persist for some hours without much change, or it may get better quickly.

The seriousness of croup is that it may progress to total or almost total closure of the windpipe leading to asphyxiation. The doctor should be called to assess the situation in all except the mildest cases. Children with croup are best observed in hospital.

Special investigations are seldom required for croup. An Xray of the chest and the neck may be done to assess the problem and to exclude the possibility of an inhaled foreign body as the cause of the breathing difficulty.

Most important is the assessment of the child's condition and progress. Pulse rate, respiratory rate, and the degree of distress and respiratory effort must be regularly observed. If the obstruction does get worse the doctors can insert a plastic tube down into the throat and through the larynx to overcome the blockage. This is called endotracheal intubation.

If endotracheal intubation is not required when the child is first seen by the doctor, supportive treatment may be given in an attempt to ease the obstruction, while the child is being observed. Steam or cold mist may help to loosen any mucous secretions that may be collecting in the throat. Antibiotics do not help in ordinary croup, which is caused by a viral infection.

Croup will often get better during the day, only to return the next night. The whole episode may last only a few hours, or can persist on and off for days, but the obstruction seldom worsens after the first 24 hours.

Epiglottitis
This is a very severe, life-threatening form of croup. Unlike ordinary croup, epiglottitis is caused by a bacteria, haemophilus influenzae, which affects the back of the throat and rapidly progresses to obstruct the airways completely. Prompt treatment is essential. An endotracheal tube should be inserted, or a tracheostomy performed, together with intravenous antibiotics and other supportive measures.

Endotracheal tube

Laryngeal airway

Trachea

Endotracheal intubation In severe croup, where there is marked narrowing of the laryngeal airway, it may be necessary for the doctors to pass a tube through the obstruction, or to do a tracheostomy, which is making a surgical opening in the front of the windpipe and inserting a special tube.

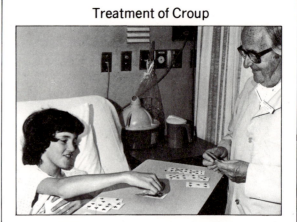

Treatment of Croup

The importance of croup from a medical point of view is that the airway may become dangerously narrowed by inflammation. The child needs careful observation, and the doctor should be consulted. Nursing the child in a humid atmosphere, provided by a steam kettle or a humidifier, helps to loosen secretions and prevent them causing further obstruction to the airway.

Pneumonia

PNEUMONIA IS AN INFECTION of the lung itself rather than just the air passages. This infection may be secondary to another problem, such as asthma, or inhaling food or a foreign body, or it may follow another infection such as measles or influenza. This secondary infection is termed bronchopneumonia. Less commonly, pneumonia results from direct infection, but this is now rare in healthy children.

The infecting organism in pneumonia is usually bacterial, but occasionally viruses and intermediary organisms called mycoplasma can invade the lungs.

The symptoms of pneumonia include coughing and a fever which varies in severity. The cough may be dry and distressing, or may be productive of sputum which is often yellow or green. Children often swallow sputum rather than spitting it out. There may also be breathlessness if the infection is extensive. Other features will depend on the particular reason for the infection, and on which organism is the infecting agent.

The doctor may find evidence of infection of the lungs on examining the chest, but if pneumonia is suspected, a chest Xray will normally be done to show the extent of the infection. If sputum is being coughed up, a sample will be sent to the laboratory for identification of the organisms causing the infection.

The child will probably be treated with antibiotics and may not, therefore, need to go into hospital. The doctor may also prescribe physiotherapy to teach the child to breathe correctly and clear the chest.

Bronchiolitis

In young babies, up to about 18 months of age, a viral lung infection called bronchiolitis sometimes occurs. The small airways become narrowed because of swelling of the lining membrane. The child wheezes and has difficulty in breathing, because of the obstructed airways, and this is sometimes severe. Skilled nursing care in hospital, and sometimes oxygen therapy and drugs, usually ensures complete recovery after a few days.

Wheezy bronchitis

With babies in the six months to two year period, wheezing may accompany colds and other infections. This is most common in babies who are overweight. The infection starts as a headcold but rapidly moves to the chest causing coughing and wheezing. Usually the baby is not particularly ill, but he may be fretful and have difficulty feeding. Occasionally, symptoms are more severe and the child requires hospitalization for a few days.

These attacks are usually diagnosed as acute or wheezy bronchitis, and are often treated with an antibiotic. Improvement occurs in a few days, but in some children these attacks of wheezy bronchitis are the first indication that the child is developing asthma.

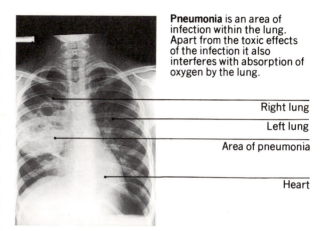

Pneumonia is an area of infection within the lung. Apart from the toxic effects of the infection it also interferes with absorption of oxygen by the lung.

Right lung

Left lung

Area of pneumonia

Heart

Chest Physiotherapy

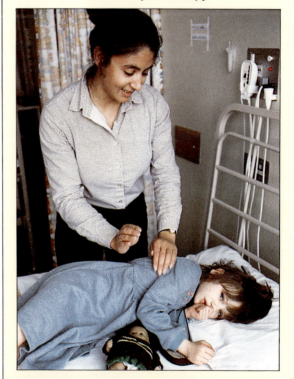

The physiotherapist aids the drainage of secretions from the lungs by positioning the child and percussing the chest and back to remove the thick mucus. The positions are varied during the treatment to enable all parts of the infected lung to be drained. In bad infections physiotherapy may be necesary several times a day.

The heart and circulation

THE ORGANS OF THE body need a constant supply of blood to provide them with the oxygen and nourishment they need to function. The heart acts as a pump to circulate the blood around the organs. The left side of the heart pumps blood rich in oxygen around the body. This blood returns to the right side of the heart with much of the oxygen used up and carrying carbon dioxide and other waste produces from the organs. The right side of the heart then pumps this blood to the lungs to pick up more oxygen and to discharge the carbon dioxide. This oxygenated blood then returns to the left side of the heart to be recirculated around the body. Blood containing oxygen is bright red in colour, blood without oxygen is dark and bluish.

The heart has a thick muscular wall and repeated contractions of this heart muscle pumps the blood around. A system of valves in the heart ensures a one-way flow.

Examination of the heart

When the doctor is examining the heart and circulation for disease, he will want to know about the symptoms

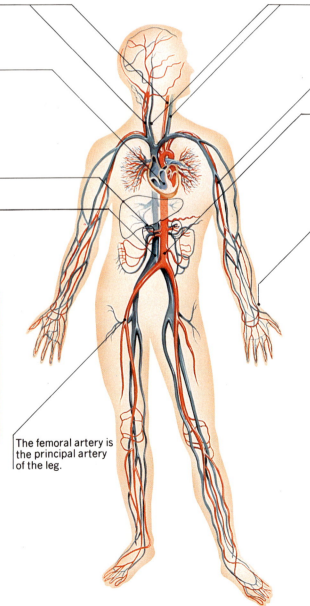

The carotid arteries go from the aorta to the head. They supply the brain with blood which carries vital oxygen and nutrients.

The heart is at the centre of the circulatory system. A network of arteries and veins enables blood to circulate around the body. Arteries carry blood away from the heart to the tissues and cells; veins carry blood from the same cells back to the heart.

Liver and kidneys

The inferior vena cava is the major vein from the lower part of the body, and carries blood returning to the right atrium from the legs, pelvis and abdomen.

The jugular veins carry the blood returning from the head on its way towards the heart.

The brachial artery is the principal artery of the arm.

The aorta is the major artery of the body. It carries all the blood pumped out of the left ventricle of the heart. It arches over the heart and then runs down the body in front of the vertebral column until it divides into two branches which go to the legs.

The radial artery is a branch of the brachial artery supplying blood to the forearm and part of the hand. It runs close to the surface of the wrist and is the artery we feel when taking the pulse.

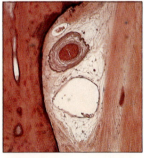

Arteries carry blood away from the heart. Their walls are extremely strong which enable them to withstand the pressure of the blood being pushed along them. Arteries and veins both have the same three basic layers but the wall of an artery is much thicker because it contains far more muscle and elastic tissue. In the photograph above the artery is shown at the top with the vein below.

The femoral artery is the principal artery of the leg.

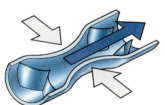

Veins carry blood to the heart. They have valves which allow blood to flow one way only. In the diagram above the blue arrow indicates the flow of blood through the vein. As the pockets of the valves fill with blood they are forced together to prevent any backflow of blood. The grey arrows indicate muscular pressure on the walls of the vein. When the muscles contract blood is forced through the valves towards the heart.

How the heart works

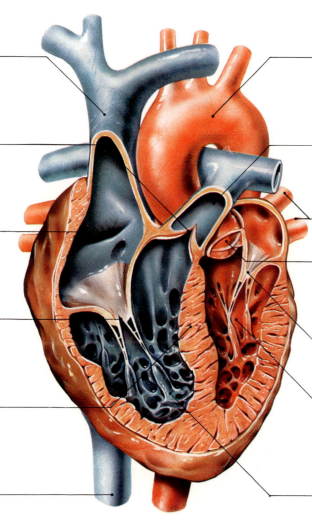

The superior vena cava carries blood from the upper part of the body to the heart.

The pulmonary valve has three flaps which open to let blood flow from the right ventricle and then close to stop it returning.

The right atrium receives deoxygenated blood from the superior and inferior vena cavae.

The tricuspid valve enables blood to flow from the right atrium into the right ventricle.

The ventricular septum separates the right and left ventricles.

The inferior vena cava carries blood from the lower part of the body to the heart.

The aorta is the main artery of the body and carries blood from the heart to the body. It receives oxygenated blood from the left ventricle.

The pulmonary artery carries blood from the heart to the lungs for oxygenation.

The pulmonary veins carry oxygenated blood from the lungs to the heart.

The aortic valve controls the flow of blood from the left ventricle into the aorta.

The mitral valve controls the flow of blood from the left atrium to the left ventricle.

The left ventricle pumps blood into the aorta and around the body.

The right ventricle receives blood from the right atrium and pumps it into the pulmonary artery.

The heart must be constantly at work to maintain the circulation of the blood which distributes oxygen and nutrients around the body, and removes waste products. Each beat of the heart pumps out some blood into the circulation. From the left side of the heart this goes to the body, and from the right to the lungs.

On each side the heart has an atrium and a ventricle. The atrium collects blood returning to the heart, and then contracts, pumping the blood into the ventricle.

The heart wall consists of special muscle which repeatedly contracts and relaxes throughout life. There are valves within the heart which ensure a one way flow of blood.

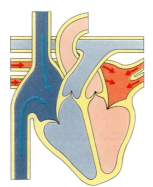

1. Between contractions of the heart blood flows into the right and left atria.

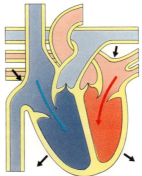

2. With atrial contraction blood is pumped into the ventricles. The ventricles increase in size as the blood enters.

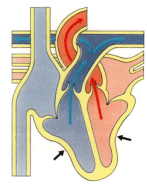

3. On contraction of the ventricle the atrioventricular valve closes, the valves at the exit to the heart (pulmonary and aortic valves) open, and blood is pumped out under pressure.

Testing blood pressure Blood pressure is measured by putting a band around the arm, and determining what pressure is required to stop the flow of blood. The blood pressure depends partly on the amount of work the heart is doing, and partly on the degree of constriction of the blood vessels.

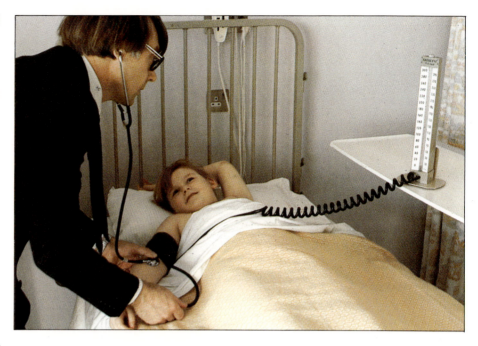

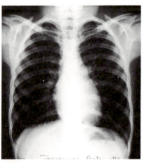

Chest Xray A chest Xray shows the size and shape of the heart. An enlarged heart signifies that at least part of it is overworking.

such as blueness of the face and breathlessness. When studying the child, the doctor will look for blueness of the lips, indicating poor oxygenation of the blood. He will feel the pulse to find out its rate and how strong it is. He will also feel the chest to identify the heart beat, and will listen to the heart with a stethoscope. When the heart is working normally the closure of the two pairs of heart valves can be heard. Any additional noises made by the heart are called murmurs.

Chest Xray. The size and shape of the heart can be seen on a chest Xray. In some forms of congenital heart disease characteristic alterations in heart shape and arrangement show up, which helps to establish a diagnosis.

Electrocardiogram. The electrocardiogram, or ECG, is a recording of the electrical activity of the heart made with recording wires attached to the arms and legs, and across the chest. It enables the heart rhythm to be studied and will indicate if parts of the heart are overworked.

Phonocardiography. Phonocardiography is a visual recording of the noises made by the heart as it contracts. The sensitivity of the recording and the fact that it can be studied slowly mean that more information can be obtained from a phonocardiogram than from listening to the heart with a stethoscope.

Echocardiography. The heart can also be studied by ultrasound. Measurement of the size of the various heart chambers, the thickness of the walls and the movement of the valves can all be made using an echocardiogram.

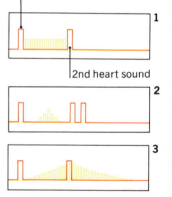

1st heart sound

2nd heart sound

1. Diagram of murmur in ventricular septal defect, showing the murmur (yellow path) is constant between first and second heart sound (red path). 2. Murmur midway between first and second sounds in atrial septal defect. The second heart sound is split. 3. Murmur in patent ductus arteriosus is both in systole (cardiac contraction) and diastole (cardiac relaxation).

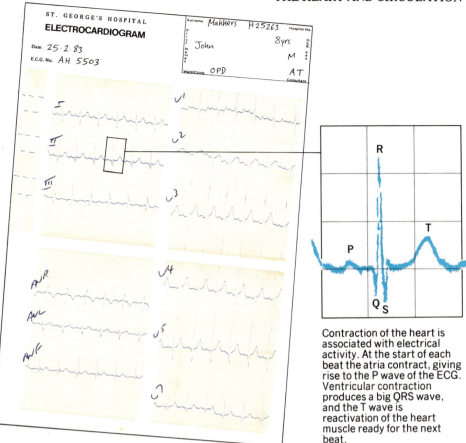

ST. GEORGE'S HOSPITAL
ELECTROCARDIOGRAM

Date: 25·2·83
E.C.G. No. AH 5503

Surname: Makhers H25263   Hospital No.
John   8yrs
M
Ward/Clinic: OPD   AT   Consultant

Electrocardiogram With each beat the heart produces a complex of electrical activity which can be amplified and recorded. This recording is called an electrocardiogram (right). It enables the doctors to study the rhythm and activity of the different parts of the heart.

Contraction of the heart is associated with electrical activity. At the start of each beat the atria contract, giving rise to the P wave of the ECG. Ventricular contraction produces a big QRS wave, and the T wave is reactivation of the heart muscle ready for the next beat.

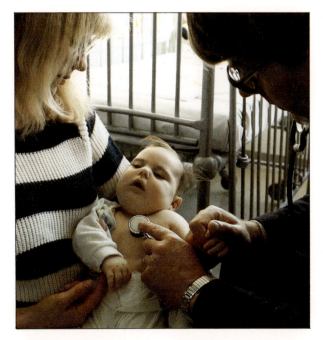

Listening to the heart As the heart beats the valves between the different chambers open and close in turn. Valve closure makes a noise which can be heard through a stethoscope. The doctor may be able to detect abnormality of valve closures. Sometimes extra noises are heard, and these are called murmurs. They may signify rapid blood flow, or narrowing of a valve, or an abnormal connection between parts of the heart.

Cardiac catheterization. In congenital heart disease, when as much information about the heart as possible has been obtained by the above tests, it may be decided to proceed to cardiac catheterization. This consists of passing a fine tube up a blood vessel from the arm or leg until it reaches the heart. Measurements of the pressure in the heart can be made, blood samples taken and special Xrays obtained during this procedure. This gives precise information about the heart, which can be used to ascertain whether any surgical treatment is necessary.

Heart Murmurs

When listening to the heart the doctor may hear a murmur, an extra sound which is present in addition to the normal sounds of the heart valve closure. Murmurs may be detected on routine medical examination, or during examination for intercurrent illness as well as in suspected cardiac disease.

Cardiac murmurs may indicate congenital heart disease with the narrowing of one of the valves of the heart, or a hole in the septum which divides the right and left sides of the heart. In children, murmurs are not usually due to disease of the heart, but are caused because the flow of blood through the heart is rapid and therefore noisy. These flow murmurs are known as innocent murmurs, as they are not indicative of disease. The doctor may be able to recognize a murmur as innocent on examining the heart, but if there is any doubt some simple investigations may be suggested. Often the doctor will merely arrange to re-examine the child when he is older, when diagnosis may be easier.

Congenital heart disease

CONGENITAL HEART DISEASE is the term used for any cardiac abnormality due to faulty development before birth. There are many different forms of congenital heart disease; some of them are serious, while others may be trivial.

The early embryological development of the heart is very complex. The heart is initially just a hollow tube, but part becomes thick and muscular and develops into the ventricles which pump the blood around the circulation. The other part has a thinner wall and forms the atria, which collect the blood returning to the heart and direct it into the ventricles. The heart becomes divided into right and left by the formation of a septum, and valves develop between the atria and ventricles and at the outlets of the heart, to ensure a one-way flow of blood. All these developmental changes occur in the first three months following conception, and if anything goes wrong then congenital heart disease can result.

Before birth the blood is not oxygenated by the lungs and the circulation to the lungs is by-passed by a special artery, the ductus arteriosus. At birth the lungs expand with the first breath and blood from the right side of the heart begins to circulate through them. The ductus arteriosus normally closes and becomes obliterated shortly after birth. Occasionally it persists and results in another form of congenital heart disease, patent ductus arteriosus. If there is persistence of a patent ductus arteriosus surgery will be required to tie the artery, which is important in foetal life, but causes overwork for the heart if it fails to close after birth.

Changes in the circulation at birth. Before birth the lungs of the foetus do not function and therefore oxygen is supplied to the foetus from the placenta via the umbilical vein. Only a small amount of blood needs to be pumped into the lungs of the foetus so there are two holes or by-passes in the heart which enable blood to avoid the lungs. These are called the ductus arteriosus and the foramen ovale (see top right).

Immediately after birth the baby becomes dependent on the lungs, rather than the placenta, for oxygen. The lungs expand and the flow of blood through them increases. The ductus arteriosus and the foramen ovale, which acted as by-passes, are no longer needed and they close up so that circulation is altered (see bottom right).

Blood flow through ductus arteriosus

To lungs

From lungs

Blood flow through foramen ovale

From body tissues and from placenta

Aorta

To lungs

From lungs

To body tissues and placenta

To lungs

From lungs

Aorta

To lungs

From lungs

RA

LA

RV

LV

From body tissues

To body tissues

Blue: deoxygenated blood
Red: oxygenated blood
Purple: mixed blood
RA: right atrium
RV: right ventricle
LV: left ventricle
LA: left atrium

Disorders of the heart at birth

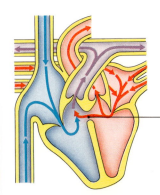

Ventricular septal defect

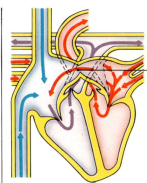

Atrial septal defect

Ventricular septal defect is the commonest form of congenital heart disease. The septum between the right and left ventricles fails to develop completely. This leaves a hole and blood flows from the left to right sides of the heart, meaning that more blood than usual has to be pumped around the lungs. This is one form of the so-called 'hole in the heart' condition. The size of the hole is very variable; small

holes cause few problems apart from producing a murmur, and these often close spontaneously during childhood. Larger holes, ventricular septal defects, cause some strain on the heart, and heart surgery to repair the defect may be needed.

Atrial septal defect is a hole in the septum between left and right at atrial level. This also leads to blood flowing from left to right sides of the heart and extra blood needs to be pumped around the lungs. Atrial septal defects may be detected if the characteristic murmur is heard during routine medical examination. They seldom cause trouble in childhood, but surgery may be required to prevent

trouble developing in the heart or lungs in adult life.

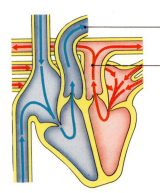

Aorta

Pulmonary artery

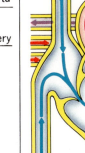

Aorta

Ductus arteriosus

Pulmonary artery

Transposition of the great vessels is one form of the 'blue baby' condition. The heart is malformed in development so that little of the blood gets oxygenated by the lungs. The babies are observed to be blue and listless from birth, and formerly many of them died. They need urgent cardiac investigation and treatment. Surgery to correct the problem is

difficult, but is often very successful. There are other forms of congenital heart disease where failure to oxygenate the blood properly leads to a child having a blue appearance. This is because deoxygenated blood is circulating around the body.

Patent ductus arteriosus is a condition which occurs when the ductus arteriosus which connects the pulmonary artery and the aorta fails to close shortly after birth. This means that blood passes from the aorta into the pulmonary artery and the heart has to overwork to compensate. If the diagnosis is made early, the defect can be closed with drug treatment. In other cases an operation to

close the duct is carried out before the child is five.

Stenosis of one of the heart valves may occur as a developmental abnormality, and consists of narrowing of the valve which partially obstructs the flow of blood.

Blood and blood diseases

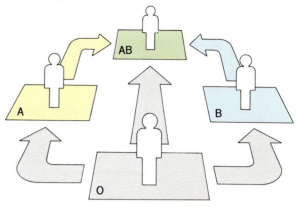

THE CIRCULATORY SYSTEM is the major transport system of the body. The blood is in continuous motion due to the pumping of the heart, and it carries oxygen from the lungs to the tissues, and carbon dioxide back to the lungs. It also transports nutrients and hormones around the body and waste products to the kidneys.

Although the blood is fluid it contains large numbers of red and white blood cells, and other small particles called platelets. The function of the red blood cells, or erythrocytes, is to transport oxygen around the body and to help in the elimination of carbon dioxide. There are enormous numbers of red cells in the body; each millilitre of blood contains about five million. The red cells are formed in the bone marrow, and each has an individual life span of three to four months. The white cells, or leucocytes, have a major role in combating infection. They are carried around the body by the blood, but can leave the circulation anywhere there is infection, and mount a defence against the invading organisms.

The platelets, or thrombocytes, are particles smaller than the red and white blood cells, which play a vital role in blood clotting. Whenever a blood vessel is cut or broken, the platelets initiate the formation of a blood clot to prevent excessive blood loss. Blood diseases may involve red cells, white cells, or the clotting process.

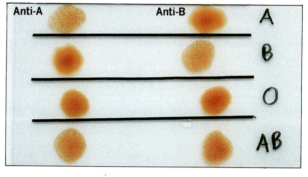

Blood tests

In suspected blood disease, the doctor will order blood tests in order to examine the appearance of the cells under a microscope. A haematologist will measure the number and size of the red and white cells, and the blood platelets. Much of the counting is now automated, using an electronic counter. Sometimes it is also necessary to look at some bone marrow to see the appearance of the blood-forming cells. Usually a sample is removed from the bone of the pelvis with a large needle, under a general or local anaesthetic.

There are several systems of blood grouping. The so-called ABO system and the rhesus system are of importance for blood transfusion. People with blood group O can only safely receive a blood donation from another O donor, but O blood can be given to individuals of blood groups O, A, B and AB. O is therefore known as a universal donor (see diagram above). Persons of blood group AB, the rarest group, can safely receive blood from individuals of groups O, A, B and AB. *(See also Blood groups and Rhesus incompatibility in the glossary).*

Cross matching of blood to make sure donor and recipient are compatible is very important. Both the ABO and rhesus groups have to be compatible for a safe blood transfusion. Blood group compatibility can be tested quite simply by putting two drops of blood on a glass plate and adding Anti-A antibodies to one and Anti-B antibodies to the other. Anti-A coalesces the cells of groups B and AB. Group O cells are not coalesced by either antibody. If the blood sample clumps then the blood is not compatible. The diagram above shows Anti-A and Anti-B serum with blood cells of different groups.

Blood clotting If the blood did not clot after injury even trivial wounds could cause dangerous loss of blood. However, it is essential that blood remains fluid within the blood vessels. Injured tissue releases substances called thromboplastins which start the clotting process. Blood platelets adhere to the edge of the wound and clotting factors in the blood are activated. These activated clotting factors induce fibrinogen, a protein dissolved in the blood, to be converted to fibrin — an insoluble complex of fibres which, together with entrapped platelets, forms the blood clot. The clot prevents further bleeding, and subsequently shrinks and forms a firm plug in the damaged blood vessel.

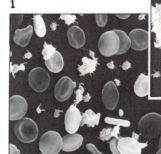

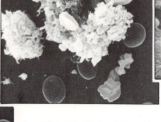

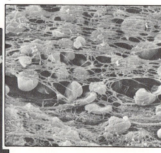

1. When first shed blood is fluid, containing red cells, white cells and platelets.
2. The platelets clump together in response to injury and release thromboplastin.
3. Thromboplastin induces the clotting factors in the blood plasma to become solid and fibrous, and the blood clot is formed.

Anaemia

The major function of the red blood cells is to transport oxygen around the body. They contain haemoglobin, a red iron-containing substance which reacts with oxygen to form a compound called oxyhaemoglobin. In the lungs haemoglobin picks up oxygen, and this is then released in the body tissues. The bone marrow makes haemoglobin within newly formed red blood cells to replace the old cells which have been destroyed in the circulation.

Anaemia occurs when the blood does not contain enough haemoglobin. Mild anaemia does not cause any symptoms, but if more severe, the ability of the blood to carry oxygen is impaired. This may give rise to breathlessness on exertion, general lethargy, and paleness.

There are many causes of anaemia. It may be due to iron deficiency leading to an inability to form haemoglobin, to blood loss from injury or internal bleeding, to excessive red cell destruction by disease, or to an inherited abnormality of red blood cells. In childhood dietary iron deficiency is the most common cause of anaemia.

Iron deficiency anaemia

There are only small amounts of iron in the diet, mainly in meat and green vegetables. At birth a baby usually has sufficient body stores of iron to suffice for the first few months of life without needing dietary iron. Milk contains virtually no iron so these stores are important. If mixed feeding is not established from about six months old, dietary iron deficiency may result, usually around the age of ten to eighteen months. After this time the iron demand is less as growth is less rapid. The diet is likely to contain adequate amounts to prevent anaemia and to replace body stores.

Low birth weight babies have very little stored iron in the body when they are born, and they need routine iron supplements to prevent anaemia in infancy.

Iron deficiency anaemia can be diagnosed on a simple blood test, and treated effectively by giving iron-enriched medicine. If the cause of the anaemia is dietary inadequacy of iron the diet should be modified to prevent a recurrence when the iron medicine is discontinued.

Although most common in toddlers, dietary iron deficiency can occur at other stages in childhood.

Sickle cell anaemia

Sickle cell anaemia is an inherited form of anaemia which affects people originally of West African descent. In sickle cell anaemia, the haemoglobin molecule is abnormal and because of this the red cells become distorted in shape, and are destroyed more rapidly than

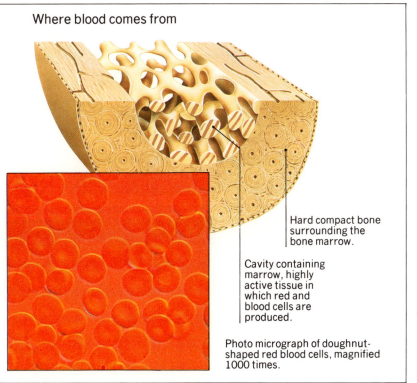

Where blood comes from

The red blood cells and many of the white blood cells are formed in the bone marrow (right), particularly the marrow inside the pelvis, vertebrae and sternum. The red cells (see enlargement, right) are formed by division of precursor cells to give new cells which each undergo a maturation process and gradually synthesise haemoglobin. When the cells contain a full amount of haemoglobin (the red pigment which binds and transports oxygen) they are released into the circulation. In this way oxygen is transported around the body in the bloodstream. In a similar way the granulocyte white blood cells are formed by maturation of precursor cells in the bone marrow.

In suspected blood disease the doctor may arrange for a bone marrow test to be done. A small amount of marrow is sucked out through a needle from the pelvis, under a general or local anaesthetic. This sample of marrow can then be stained and studied under the microscope.

Hard compact bone surrounding the bone marrow.

Cavity containing marrow, highly active tissue in which red and blood cells are produced.

Photo micrograph of doughnut-shaped red blood cells, magnified 1000 times.

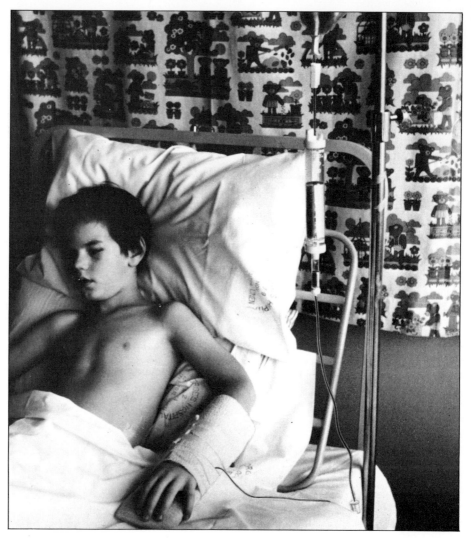

Blood transfusion is required to replace serious blood loss due to an accident or an operation. It may also be used for the treatment of some forms of anaemia. Blood has to be carefully cross-matched to make sure it is compatible with the recipient's own blood.

usual in the body. The distorted cells are crescent shaped when seen through a microscope — hence the name sickle cell disease.

Children with sickle cell disease are always moderately anaemic, but this does not usually cause significant symptoms. Of more importance, is the fact that the distorted red cells can, on occasions, cause blockage of small blood vessels and subsequent damage to tissue deprived of oxygen and nutrients. The damaged tissue gives rise to pain which may be severe. Painful episodes can affect the abdomen, chest or limbs. They usually settle in a few days, but if bone is involved, they may take much longer to subside.

Painful episodes are more likely to occur if circulation becomes sluggish due to cold, so children should be dressed warmly in winter. They may also occur during treatment for other diseases. Children with sickle cell disease are more susceptible to infection.

There is no curative treatment for sickle cell disease. Supplements of folic acid, a vitamin, help to prevent the anaemia becoming too severe, and ANALGESICS will be needed for the painful episodes. Many young children are also given regular penicillin to prevent serious infection.

If, for any reason, the affected child should need an anaesthetic, the doctor must be told about the sickle cell disease.

People who have one gene for sickle cell disease, and one gene for normal haemoglobin, have a mild anaemia, but seldom have other symptoms, and they may be unaware that they are carriers of the sickle cell gene. This is known as sickle cell trait.

If two parents both have the trait there is a 25 per cent risk of any child of theirs having sickle cell disease, and on average, another 50 per cent of their children will have the trait.

Thalassaemia

Thalassaemia is an inherited form of anaemia principally affecting people of Mediterranean, African or Asian origin. There are two forms of the disease — minor and major. Thalassaemia minor occurs when an individual has inherited one thalassaemia gene and one for normal haemoglobin. Thalassaemia major is when the abnormal gene is inherited from both parents.

With thalassaemia major there is profound anaemia due to an inability to form normal haemoglobin. Without regular transfusions these children die in infancy or early childhood.

In thalassaemia minor there is mild to moderate

anaemia, but it is compatible with a full active life. If two parents both have the minor disease there is a high (25 per cent) risk of any child having thalassaemia major. In recent years intrauterine blood testing has been introduced in special centres so that the couple can be offered an abortion of any affected foetus. This has enabled some couples to have children without the fear of the major disease.

Leukaemia

Leukaemia is a disease in which many of the normal cells of the bone marrow are replaced by abnormal cells called blast cells. These blast cells are abnormal precursors of white blood cells and they may infiltrate other organs such as the liver, spleen and glands, as well as the bone marrow.

There are several different forms of leukaemia but the type that is most common in childhood is called acute lymphoblastic leukaemia. Fortunately this is the form that is most responsive to treatment. The outlook in childhood leukaemia has changed dramatically in recent years. Nearly all patients have benefitted substantially from treatment, and many are completely cured.

The symptoms of leukaemia are mainly due to loss of the normal blood forming cells, which have been suppressed by the blast cells in the bone marrow. The affected child may become pale and weak from anaemia, prone to infection due to lack of normal white cells, or develop bruising of the skin or bleeding from the gums because of a shortage of blood platelets. These symptoms usually develop fairly quickly and the diagnosis is usually made within a week or two. On examining the child the doctor may note anaemia, infection or enlarged lymph glands or other organs. If he suspects leukaemia, he will order a blood test and a bone marrow examination.

Treatment consists of blood transfusion if the anaemia is marked and antibiotics if infection is present, together with a variety of anti-leukaemic drugs. Usually within a few weeks the child improves, and the blood

---

Treatment of leukaemia in childhood

When leukaemia has been diagnosed in childhood the doctors do various tests of the blood and bone marrow to find out which sort of leukaemia is present. The commonest form of leukaemia in childhood is acute lymphoblastic leukaemia (ALL), which is also the sort that responds best to treatment.

Drug treatment is started with anti-leukaemic drugs such as vincristine and steroids to make the disease go into remission. During this period, which may last for several weeks, supportive treatment with transfusions of whole blood or platelets, and with antibiotics may be needed.

The next phase of treatment is consolidating and maintaining this remission. As well as drugs treatment with Xrays to the head is usually given during the consolidation phase. This prevents subsequent leukaemia infiltration of the central nervous system.

After two or three years of maintenance treatment, many patients are able to discontinue drug therapy. Permanent cure is obtained in at least 60% of children with acute lymphoblastic leukaemia. In other forms of leukaemia in childhood, useful remission can usually be achieved, but long term results are not yet as good as in acute lymphoblastic leukaemia.

---

tests and bone marrow become normal. This is called going into remission. This remission is then consolidated by continuing treatment for another two or three years, using several different drugs and often Xray therapy.

After a period of consolidation is over, it is usually possible to discontinue treatment without the disease relapsing, although the child should continue to be observed for some time to make sure there is no reappearance of the disease.

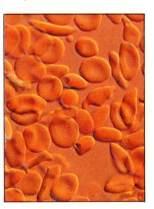 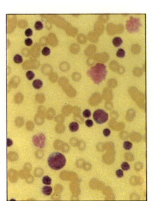

These illustrations show blood films as seen through the microscope. They are stained so that the red cells look red, and the white cells mauve. The normal red cells are round discs (far left). In sickle cell anaemia the red cells appear distorted (middle). In leukaemia (right) there is an excess of white blood cells.

Diabetes

DIABETES IS A CONDITION in which the body is unable to make enough of the hormone insulin to meet its requirements. Insulin is a vital agent in enabling the body to utilize the energy it gets from the food it eats, particularly from carbohydrates. During digestion these carbohydrate foods (sugar and starch) are converted into glucose and absorbed into the body.

Insulin is required for this glucose to be used by the body, and it is secreted by the pancreas. The insulin is then released into the bloodstream in a controlled way so that just the right amount is available, depending on the level of glucose in the blood.

With diabetes the pancreas does not produce enough insulin and, to stay healthy, children with this disease have to be given regular injections of insulin. There is another form of diabetes occurring in middle-aged and elderly people which does not always require insulin treatment, but can be treated by diet and tablets instead.

Diabetic children, however, have to have injections of insulin.

If there is a lack of insulin, as in diabetes, glucose cannot be used for energy. As a result the amount of the glucose in the blood becomes too high, and some is excreted in the urine. Much more urine than usual is passed to get rid of this excess glucose, and this causes the patient to become thirsty. Because the body cannot use glucose effectively for energy, fat is used instead, and substances called ketones are formed which can build up in the body and have harmful effects. This condition is called diabetic ketosis, and it may progress to coma if the child is not treated.

The cause of diabetes is not known, but it does sometimes run in families. Once it has developed it is present for life, and regular injections of insulin will always be required. The child will have to be on a diet regulating the amount of carbohydrate foods eaten. It is

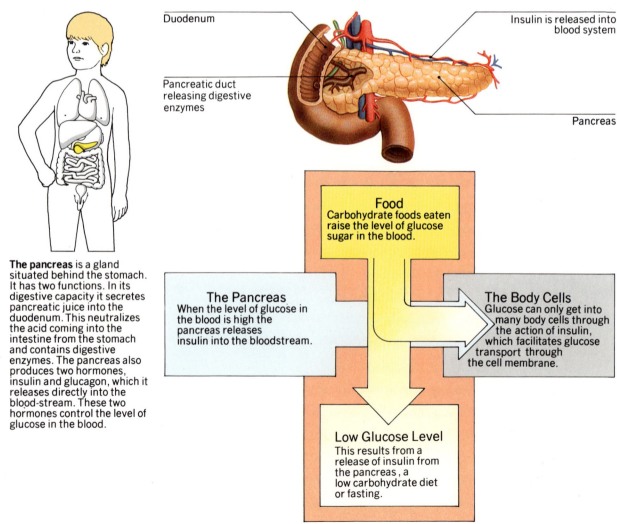

Duodenum

Pancreatic duct releasing digestive enzymes

Insulin is released into blood system

Pancreas

The pancreas is a gland situated behind the stomach. It has two functions. In its digestive capacity it secretes pancreatic juice into the duodenum. This neutralizes the acid coming into the intestine from the stomach and contains digestive enzymes. The pancreas also produces two hormones, insulin and glucagon, which it releases directly into the blood-stream. These two hormones control the level of glucose in the blood.

Food
Carbohydrate foods eaten raise the level of glucose sugar in the blood.

The Pancreas
When the level of glucose in the blood is high the pancreas releases insulin into the bloodstream.

The Body Cells
Glucose can only get into many body cells through the action of insulin, which facilitates glucose transport through the cell membrane.

Low Glucose Level
This results from a release of insulin from the pancreas, a low carbohydrate diet or fasting.

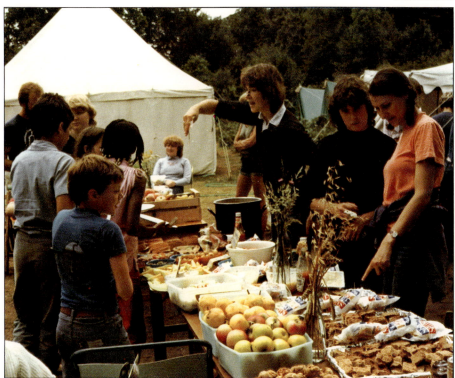

Following a diabetic diet need not be tedious. The children shown on the right are at a picnic at a diabetic camp. Each child has a card indicating the number of units (carbohydrates) they are allowed for each meal. With the help of dietitians they are able to choose an appetizing meal containing the correct amount of carbohydrates, protein and roughage. *(See also special diets, page 30).*

important to control the amount of glucose in the blood so that it is neither too high nor too low, and regular urine tests or blood tests will be needed to check how well the condition is being controlled.

The aim of treatment in diabetes is to educate the child and the family to control the condition themselves, so that they can be independent of doctors and nurses, apart from occasional visits to an outpatient clinic.

From about the age of eight children can learn to give their own injections, although for a few years the dose will need to be checked by an adult. Urine tests can be done regularly at home to get an indication of how effective the control of diabetes is. The child and adult have to learn the symptoms which suggest that the level of glucose in the blood is too low. They are hunger, sweating, weakness or feeling faint and they should be treated immediately by eating glucose or sugar lumps. Every diabetic on insulin should carry sugar or glucose at all times.

Dietary needs have to be learnt, so that the child gets the right balance of carbohydrate fat and protein foods. The carbohydrate is best taken as starch rather than as sugar, and a high intake of dietary fibre helps to maintain steady levels of glucose in the blood.

Diabetic children are particularly prone to infection if the disease is not well controlled. Any infection, particularly gastroenteritis where there is excess fluid loss, is liable to upset the control of the disease, and hospital admission may be necessary. There are also long term complications with diabetes including eye disease, heart disease, and problems with the arteries. These complications are not seen in children because they take many years to develop, but control of the disease in childhood helps to prevent the onset of problems relating to diabetes in later life.

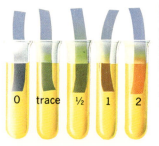

If a child has diabetes the level of glucose in his urine should be tested daily. The test tubes (left) show the levels of urinary glucose concentration in the blood. The level should read negative. If every urine test contains some glucose, control is not ideal.

0   trace   ½   1   2

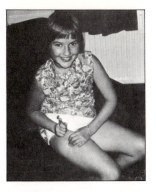

The child (left) is injecting herself in the front of the thigh. Suitable sites are the outer side of the upper arm, the outer sides and fronts of the thighs, the upper parts of the buttocks and the front of the abdomen. It is important to keep changing the injection sites so that a different place is used each day. If the same place is used repeatedly painful lumps form which may stop insulin being properly absorbed.

Over-dependence on parents, and emotional problems, are common in teenage diabetics. Adolescence tends to be a time of insecurity and injections for diabetes, and clinic attendance provide additional stress. Furthermore, the realization that they have an incurable disease, that diabetes will impose some limitations on their lifestyle, may provoke emotional reactions. With support and patience, these problems can be dealt with. Many children are helped by attending diabetic 'camps' where they mix with other children who are also facing the problems of growing up with diabetes.

The digestive system

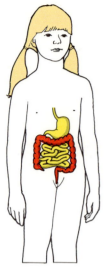

Investigation of the digestive system When disease of the digestive system is suspected the doctor may want to do some investigations. Ordinary Xrays of the abdomen show the outline of the stomach and intestines, but if a detailed study is needed, barium investigations are required.

Barium swallow and meal Barium salts inhibit the passage of Xrays, so that when a barium meal is swallowed, and the body is examined by Xrays, the digestive system is outlined. First of all the oesophagus (gullet) shows up, then the stomach, and then the barium goes on through the intestines (yellow, above). Hiatus hernia, pyloric stenosis and intestinal disease may be diagnosed in this way.

Barium enema For diseases of the lower end of the bowel, such as Hirschsprung's disease, or ulcerative colitis, it may be necessary to give an enema containing barium to demonstrate the lesion (red, above).

THE DIGESTIVE SYSTEM includes the mouth, the oesophagus (gullet), the stomach, the small intestine, the large intestine (also known as the colon), and the rectum. When food is eaten it is chewed and mixed with saliva and then passed through the oesophagus into the stomach. The digestive process starts in the stomach, where the food is broken down by acid and digestive enzymes. Gradually the stomach contents are passed into the small intestine. Here they are mixed with bile from the liver and pancreatic juice which further help in breaking the food down into a form in which it can be absorbed.

Absorption of food takes place in the small intestine; water is aborbed in the large intestine. The inabsorbable food material and digestive wastes form the faeces, which collect in the rectum until defaecation.

Disease of the digestive system may give rise to varied symptoms including poor appetite, vomiting, abdominal pain, diarrhoea, constipation or weight loss. Poor appetite and consequent loss of weight are often signs of digestive disease, influenced by the state of the digestive tract and by psychological factors. Weight may also be lost if the food is not absorbed properly, even when adequate amounts are eaten.

Abdominal pain may come from disorder of the digestive tract or from other organs within the abdominal cavity such as the kidneys, bladder, or liver. Pain which originates in other parts of the body may also be felt in the abdomen. This is discussed more fully later on page 100.

Vomiting is a mechanism for emptying the stomach. It can occur because too much has been eaten, or because something noxious has been eaten. It occurs if there is any obstruction of the digestive tract. Sometimes, as in motion sickness or with anxiety, the cause may be the nervous system.

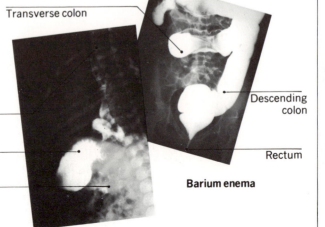

Oesophagus

Hiatus hernia

Stomach

Transverse colon

Descending colon

Rectum

Barium enema

Barium meal

Everyone needs food to maintain the health of his or her body. In order for food to be utilized, it must be broken down into molecules small enough to be absorbed. This takes place through the digestive process.

Food is chewed, mixed with saliva, swallowed and passed through the oesophagus into the stomach.

The stomach mixes the food with acid and digestive enzymes.

Gradually the stomach contents are passed into the small intestine. Here, juice from the pancreas, bile from the liver, and digestive enzymes from the intestinal wall break down large molecules in the food into smaller units.

Absorption of food into the bloodstream takes place in the small intestine through the villi. From here it is ferried to the liver. Water is absorbed in large intestine.

The kidneys filter the blood and make urine from waste chemicals and water.

Unabsorbed food, including dietary fibre, is turned into faeces which collect in the rectum and are excreted through the anus.

The liver receives the dissolved products of digestion such as amino acids, fatty acids, glucose and vitamins and metabolizes these products for transport by the blood.

The blood carries the nutrients derived from food to all the cells of the body.

The nutrients diffuse into the cells from the body. Once there, they are used according to their nutritional value.

The digestive process

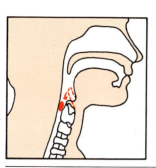

The mouth is the beginning of the digestive system. It breaks food down by chewing with the teeth and tongue. To make swallowing easy, it lubricates food with saliva. It also modifies the temperature of food. Food passes into the oesophagus, a muscular narrow tube (above), where powerful muscular contractions squeeze it into the stomach.

Duodenum

The pancreas is located behind the stomach. It produces juices which pass along the pancreatic duct into the duodenum. These juices help break down carbohydrates, proteins and fats.

Ascending colon

Rectum

Oesophagus

The liver performs many functions in the body. In its digestive system it secretes a bitter, greenish fluid called bile. Bile is stored in the gall bladder, a reservoir inside the liver, and is released periodically into the duodenum where it breaks down fatty foods.

The stomach stores food before releasing it into the duodenum. It churns and squeezes food, turning it into chyme (semi-liquid food), partly digests it and releases acids which kill off harmful bacteria.

Descending colon

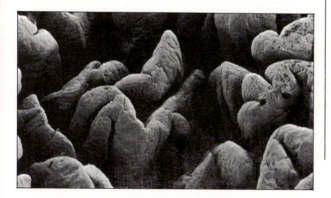

The small intestine is divided into the duodenum, jejunum and ileum. It is where the major part of both digestion and absorption takes place. Once food has been broken down by digestion, it is absorbed into the bloodstream. This takes place through millions of tiny villi (left) which line the intestinal wall (right).

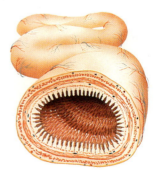

Vomiting in infancy

SOME REGURGITATION OR possetting of milk after a feed, often on bringing up the wind, is very common in babies. This does not constitute vomiting, in which a large part of the stomach contents are expelled, and is not usually of medical significance.

In the newborn period, if a baby vomits, consideration has to be given to the possibility that a congenital abnormality giving rise to obstruction of the digestive tract may be present. Such obstruction can occur at different levels. The oesophagus is sometimes malformed and may connect with the lungs, the so-called tracheo-oesophageal fistula. Babies with this deformity cough and splutter when given their first feed. The upper small intestine may be blocked due to a congenital defect, duodenal atresia, or lower down there may be an imperforate anus. Xrays are very helpful in diagnosing digestive tract obstruction; once diagnosed they can be corrected surgically with good results.

Other causes of vomiting in the newborn period include intercurrent infection, and cerebral irritation due to a difficult delivery. Sometimes blood and mucus swallowed at the time of delivery can cause gastric irritation and lead to vomiting.

Vomiting which starts later in infancy could be caused by infection. It can be a feature of gastroenteritis, urinary infection, meningitis, septicaemia or other infection. Detection of the site of the infection may not be easy, and often requires microbiological investigation of specimens and swabs. The doctor will start antibiotic treatment without waiting for the results as infections can progress rapidly in infants.

Feeding difficulties in infancy are occasionally associated with vomiting, but other causes of vomiting to be considered are *pyloric stenosis* and *hiatus hernia*.

Pyloric Stenosis

This condition in infancy results from an overgrowth of the muscle which surrounds the lower end of the stomach. This muscular overdevelopment causes progressive narrowing of the stomach outlet. When the obstruction becomes severe, little milk can leave the stomach to enter the intestine, and it is vomited instead. Although not all the factors which contribute to the development of pyloric stenosis are known, it often shows a familial tendency. Boys are more likely to be affected than girls, and first-born children seem to be at special risk.

The onset of vomiting in pyloric stenosis is usually between three and six weeks of age, during or just after a feed. The attacks are usually forceful and as they continue the baby begins to lose weight and becomes hungry and unhappy all the time. Bowel actions become less frequent. If diagnosis and treatment are delayed the baby may become depleted of water and essential minerals as well as deprived of nourishment.

The doctor may be able to detect the swelling of the overgrown pyloric muscle by feeling the abdomen during a feed. Doctors call this a pyloric tumour, but it is only an overgrowth of muscle, and not a tumourous growth in the usual meaning of the word. Sometimes an Xray is needed to make the diagnosis. The treatment of pyloric stenosis is surgical; a cut is made through the overgrown pyloric muscle, which relieves the obstruction. Normal feeding can be resumed within hours of the operation and there are seldom any further problems.

Hiatus Hernia

When the stomach is full of milk, regurgitation is normally prevented by closure of the cardiac sphincter at

---

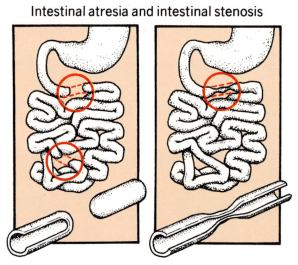

Intestinal atresia and intestinal stenosis

Intestinal atresia An atresia is a developmental anomaly with the failure of formation of part of the body. Atresia of the intestine is where a segment of the gut has not formed properly, causing a blockage. The most common site of intestinal atresia in babies is in the duodenum.

Intestinal stenosis Stenosis means a narrowing of one of the body structures. Intestinal stenosis may occur as an abnormality of development or be secondary to some other disease, such as Crohn's Disease.

Pyloric stenosis

Pyloric stenosis is a narrowing of the pylorus, the muscular tube at the end of the stomach, The wall of the pylorus thickens so that the baby's feed cannot pass into the intestine from the stomach. This means that the stomach cannot empty normally. It therefore becomes distended and the baby will vomit repeatedly after feeds. The baby will eventually lose weight and, if not treated, may become seriously dehydrated.

The baby's feed is passing normally through the stomach outlet (1). The wall of the pylorus thickens and prevents the feed leaving the stomach (2).

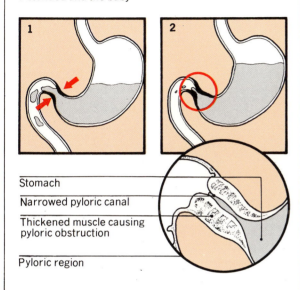

Stomach

Narrowed pyloric canal

Thickened muscle causing pyloric obstruction

Pyloric region

Hiatus hernia

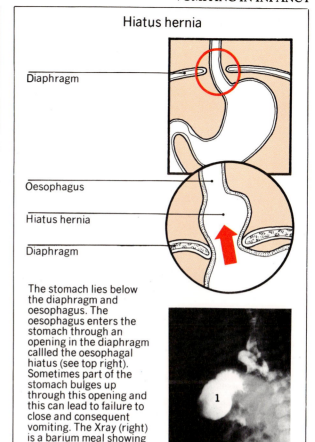

Diaphragm

Oesophagus

Hiatus hernia

Diaphragm

The stomach lies below the diaphragm and oesophagus. The oesophagus enters the stomach through an opening in the diaphragm callled the oesophagal hiatus (see top right). Sometimes part of the stomach bulges up through this opening and this can lead to failure to close and consequent vomiting. The Xray (right) is a barium meal showing a hiatus hernia (1).

the lower end of the oesophagus. As it passes from thorax to abdomen, the oesophagus goes through a hole in the diaphragm known as the oesophageal hiatus. Occasionally this hiatus is larger than normal and part of the stomach can move up into it. This is known as a hiatus hernia. When this happens the working of the cardiac sphincter is upset and regurgitation, or reflux, of gastric contents up into the oesophagus may occur. Reflux is most marked on lying down, and can lead to vomiting of much of the stomach contents.

A baby with hiatus hernia will vomit or regurgitate frequently, especially on lying down. Symptoms may start immediately after birth, or may not be noted for a week or two.

If the vomiting is marked, there will also be poor weight gain. Occasionally, because stomach acids inflame the oesophageal lining, slight bleeding can occur, and anaemia may develop.

The hiatus hernia and associated reflux can be shown on Xray. Treatment is directed to nursing the baby in a more upright position and to thickening the feeds. A baby chair, which enables the infant to be nursed at an angle of about 45 degrees, will often effectively stop the reflux. To achieve a greater tilt the child needs supporting with a harness in a special chair. Thickening feeds with pureed solids, or special food additives makes reflux less likely. Symptoms of hiatus hernia gradually abate after the first few months, and have virtually disappeared by the time the child is a year old.

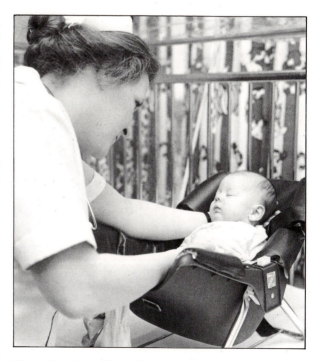

Where there is vomiting with a hiatus hernia, the baby can be nursed and fed in a sitting position in a special baby chair. This will help prevent reflux and make the baby more comfortable.

Abdominal pain

ABDOMINAL PAIN IS ONE of the most common symptoms of childhood. Although it may indicate the presence of disease, it is also a frequent symptom of anxiety and stress and sometimes occurs for no obvious reason.

The onset of abdominal pain in a child who has previously been well may indicate a digestive disturbance, possibly following something rich or unusual to eat, or overindulgence. *Constipation, urinary infections* and *appendicitis* may all be accompanied by abdominal pain.

In children abdominal pain may occur with disease elsewhere; tonsilitis and asthma can both be accompanied by tummyache, and this may occur with other infections. Severe or prolonged abdominal pain in a child who is usually healthy warrants a medical opinion.Accompanying symptoms, such as vomiting, fever or bowel disturbance, may help to elucidate the cause.

Some children get recurrent attacks of abdominal pain. This may be due to underlying disease, but usually no immediate cause is found. Disorders which may result in repeated attacks include urinary infection and obstruction, *sickle cell disease, constipation* and CROHN'S DISEASE. A medical opinion should be sought if a child has recurrent attacks of pain, particularly if they are severe; further investigations may be suggested. It is not usually necessary to consult the doctor with every bout of pain.

Recurrent abdominal pain in children is often an indication of underlying stress or anxiety. The pain may become very severe, making the child cry. It may persist for only a few minutes, or for several hours. It is usually felt in the middle of the abdomen, around the umbilicus and it can recur daily or be less frequent. Often, after a bout of abdominal pain, the child will be well for several months before there is a recurrence.

The name periodic syndrome, or abdominal migraine, is sometimes given to these bouts of abdominal pain, not associated with underlying organic disease. The child who is liable to such attacks has a particular underlying body make-up and personality, but usually there are external factors which provoke the attacks, such as stress or anxiety. Excitement or other strong emotion can bring on an attack.

It is difficult, and unnecessary, to identify an obvious precipitant for each attack, but if a child is having frequent spasms, consideration should be given to underlying problems. Children may not be aware themselves of the causes of inner tension. Stress within the family which is caused by sickness, unemployment, or marital discord, can provoke attacks, and problems at school are often at the root of the illness. There may be pressure at school because a child has a teacher he dislikes, or is experiencing difficulty with lessons. Bullying or teasing will cause anxiety which can precipitate abdominal pain, and in some children the tension inevitably associated with striving to do well in learning or written work may cause stress symptoms. Once it is realized that the attacks do not signify underlying disease, they often become easier to manage. Quiet and sympathetic support is the mainstay. If the pain is severe, the child may want to be in bed, and a hot water bottle on the tummy is soothing. Soluble aspirin or paracetamol also help with some children.

Constipation

There is a wide variation in patterns of bowel action between individuals. For some children defaecation two or three times a day is normal, while others pass stools every two or three days. To some extent the pattern of bowel action can be influenced by diet. If a child's diet contains a lot of fibre (unabsorbable roughage such as occurs in fruit and vegetables, and in breakfast cereals high in bran), the stools will tend to be soft and bulky and more frequent bowel actions are likely.Other foods, such as figs, prunes and rhubarb, tend to have a laxative effect.

In constipation the stools are hard and difficult to pass, and bowel actions become less frequent. Some children always seem to be a bit costive and they may well benefit from an increase in the amount of fibre and fruit in their diet. In other children, constipation may be an occasional happening; frequently it follows an intercurrent infection in which the appetite was temporarily depressed.

If the child becomes constipated, and has to strain, defaecation is likely to be painful. The child may become apprehensive about opening his bowels and may try and hold back. At this stage there is often refusal to sit on the potty or toilet. As a consequence, the stool is retained in the rectum and becomes even harder as more water is absorbed.

A vicious circle can soon be set up with the discomfort of constipation leading to stool retention, and therefore worse constipation. At this stage merely increasing the amount of fibre in the diet is an inadequate method of resolving the problem. Treatment with laxatives is necessary, and the cycle is broken when the regular passage of soft stools leads to a lessening of anxiety and apprehension.

Many parents and doctors are reluctant to give laxatives to children but they are necessary for severe constipation, and need to be given regularly. The aim is to achieve regular bowel action with soft stools, and then gradually reduce the laxative dose once this has been achieved.

The intermittent use of laxatives when the child is con-

Abdominal pain — making a diagnosis When the doctor is called to see a child who has abdominal pain he needs to find out as much as he can by asking questions about the child's symptoms, and by examination.

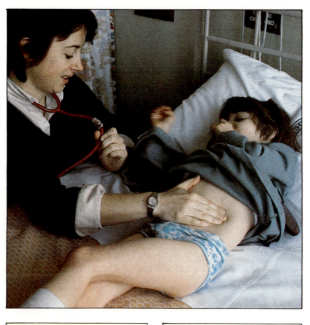

Does your child have a cold or a sore throat? Abdominal pain often complicates infection elsewhere in small children. Tonsillitis and otitis media may present like this in infancy.

When did it come on? Is this the first attack, or has it happened before, and how long has the pain been present. This will help to build up a list of possible causes.

When were the bowels last open? Constipation may cause abdominal pain, and in inflammation such as appendicitis the bowels may stop working properly.

Where is the pain? The site of the pain and whether it has moved may give important clues about which organ is involved.

What is the pain like? Colicky pains in children usually arise in the intestine. With inflammation the pain is usually continuous and made worse by movement.

Has there been vomiting or diarrhoea? Diarrhoea with abdominal pain usually indicates gastroenteritis or dysentery. Vomiting may be part of gastroenteritis or functional bowel disorder, or be due to obstruction.

Does it hurt to pass water? Painful urination, often accompanied with frequency of wanting to urinate, is very suggestive of a urinary infection.

stipated does not retrain the bowel to perform normally. There are a wide variety of suitable laxatives available. Milk of magnesia is mild and suitable for babies if the temporary addition of brown sugar to their diet is ineffective. For older children many doctors will use Lactulose syrup or a senna preparation. If a liquid preparation is used it is easy to vary the dose depending on response, gradually increasing it until the stools are soft and regular, and reducing it if they become too loose. Daily administration after breakfast is usually suitable, as most laxatives take four to six hours to take effect.

Doctors are always reluctant to use suppositories or enemas in children, but these are occasionally necessary when the constipation is so severe the laxatives are ineffective.

Once an episode of constipation has been overcome, it is important to try and prevent a recurrence. Some children seem particularly prone to recurrent bouts. A plentiful intake of fruit such as apples, oranges and prunes, vegetables high in fibre such as cabbage and greens, and bran in wholemeal bread and breakfast cereals, will help.

Faecal soiling (encopresis)
A few children with severe constipation pass small amounts of solid or liquid stool intermittently into their underclothes. This occurs because the rectum is loaded with a large faecal mass causing partial bowel obstruction and disturbance of the control of the anal sphincter. If only liquid faeces can get past the obstruction the child may mistakenly be thought to have chronic diarrhoea. Frequent faecal soiling is an indication that the child should be referred to a specialist for assessment.

Anal fissure
The passage of hard stools may lead to small tears (or fissures) in the skin around the anus. Streaks of blood on the stool are noted, and the child will complain of pain on defaecation. Soothing creams applied locally, and treatment of the constipation, are necessary to promote healing of the fissure.

Appendicitis

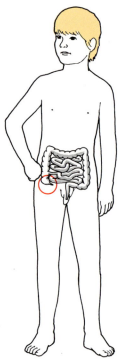

THE APPENDIX IS A narrow, blind-ended tube measuring about 3 inches which arises at the point where the small intestine joins the colon. Although it is connected to the gut it performs no digestive function in man. It does, however, sometimes become infected — the condition known as appendicitis. Infection in the appendix seldom settles down uneventfully. Usually there is a marked local reaction and pus may form inside the appendix. If not removed in time it may perforate (or burst) allowing infected material to escape into the abdominal cavity and cause PERITONITIS.

Appendicitis usually starts with abdominal pain centred around the navel (umbilicus). This is associated with malaise and loss of appetite. The pain persists, and usually gets worse for several hours. There may be vomiting, a slight temperature, and a furred tongue. Gradually the pain moves to the right side of the abdomen and the doctor looks for tenderness over the appendix when he is examining the child.

If the doctor suspects appendicitis he is likely to refer the child to a surgeon, because a definite diagnosis is not always easy to make. The doctor may order a blood count and an abdominal Xray to help in assessing the patient.

Once the diagnosis is certain arrangements are made for an operation to remove the appendix. This is usually straightforward, but may be technically difficult if there is a lot of surrounding inflammation. The appendix is cut off, the hole in the bowel wall is repaired, and the incision closed. Usually within a few days the child is ready to go home, but it may take two or three months for him to regain all his former energy. The absence of the appendix causes no problems at all, as it is known to have no significant function.

Appendicitis When the appendix becomes infected there will be abdominal pain and tenderness, slight fever, loss of appetite and maybe vomiting. The pain usually starts in the central abdomen around the umbilicus, but after a few hours moves to the right over the appendix.
The abdomen is tender to touch, particularly near the appendix.
The temperature is usually raised slightly, up to about 38.5°C/100°F.
The appetite is poor, and the tongue is usually coated with white fur. There may be an unpleasant smell to the breath.
Vomiting may occur once or twice, but is rarely persistent.

The Appendix (see right) is a narrow tubular organ arising from the junction of the small and large intestines, which looks rather like an earthworm in size and shape. It has no digestive function, but can become blocked and infected, setting up inflammation. This inflammation may cause the appendix to burst, spreading the infection more widely.

The child will be admitted to hospital as an emergency, because of abdominal pain. The appendix has to be removed by operation where there is appendicitis. The child is anaesthetised, and the skin is cleaned with an antiseptic. The skin is then covered with sterile drapes. The surgeon cuts through the skin and the abdominal wall. The incision may be over the appendix, or near the mid-line. Any bleeding has to be controlled. The appendix then has to be idenitified and freed from the membranes which hold it down. It is then tied off, held in a clamp, and cut across near the base. A stitch is placed right around the stump to seal it completely and prevent any leakage of intestinal contents. The operation is completed by repairing the abdominal wall and stitching the skin.
Within a few days of the operation the child can leave hospital, but it will be several weeks before he is fully recovered.

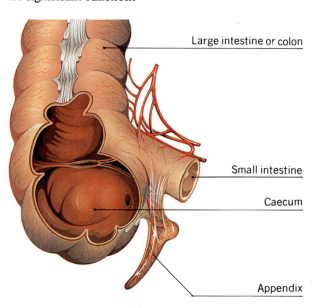

Large intestine or colon

Small intestine

Caecum

Appendix

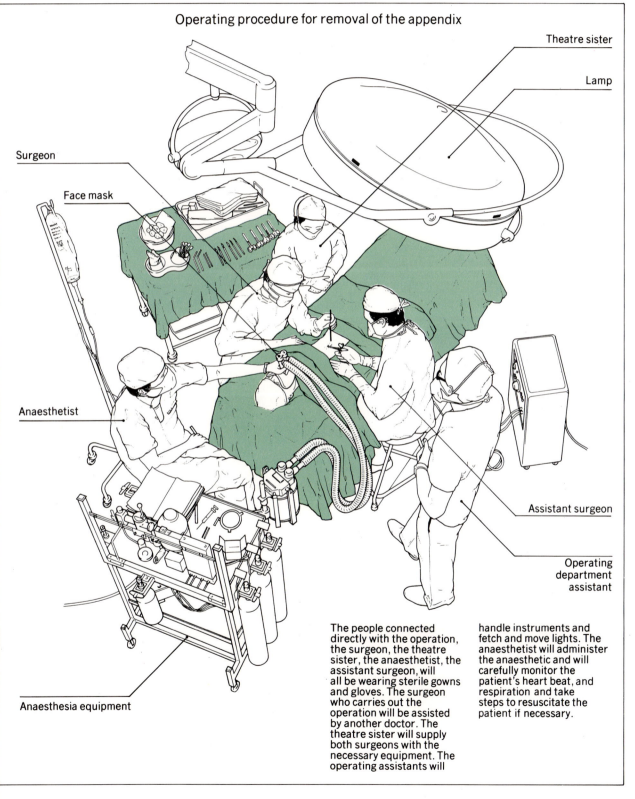

Operating procedure for removal of the appendix

Theatre sister

Lamp

Surgeon

Face mask

Anaesthetist

Assistant surgeon

Operating department assistant

Anaesthesia equipment

The people connected directly with the operation, the surgeon, the theatre sister, the anaesthetist, the assistant surgeon, will all be wearing sterile gowns and gloves. The surgeon who carries out the operation will be assisted by another doctor. The theatre sister will supply both surgeons with the necessary equipment. The operating assistants will handle instruments and fetch and move lights. The anaesthetist will administer the anaesthetic and will carefully monitor the patient's heart beat, and respiration and take steps to resuscitate the patient if necessary.

Hernias

A HERNIA (OR RUPTURE) consists of part of an internal organ protruding through a weakness in the wall of the abdominal cavity. In children sites of weakness can occur as a developmental anomaly of the abdominal wall in the groin, and in the umbilicus. Hernias in these regions are called inguinal and umbilical hernias respectively. A *hiatus hernia* is an internal hernia, where part of the stomach protrudes through a defect in the diaphragm into the chest.

Inguinal hernia

Hernias in the groin are more common in boys than in girls. In the male, during foetal development, the testicles migrate from inside the abdominal cavity into the scrotum through a passage known as the inguinal canal. The canal normally closes after the testicles have passed through, but it may remain open, forming a gap in the abdominal wall muscles through which a loop of intestines can pass.

Inguinal hernias are usually noted in infancy but can persist throughout childhood. Most frequently a lump will be noted in the groin, or extending down into the scrotum, when the child is being changed. If the child cries the hernia becomes larger and feels tense.

The inguinal canal is relatively long and narrow, and the intestine which protrudes through in an inguinal her-

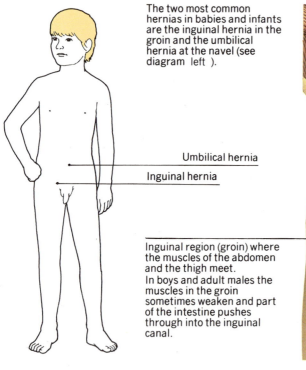

The two most common hernias in babies and infants are the inguinal hernia in the groin and the umbilical hernia at the navel (see diagram left).

Umbilical hernia

Inguinal hernia

Inguinal region (groin) where the muscles of the abdomen and the thigh meet.
In boys and adult males the muscles in the groin sometimes weaken and part of the intestine pushes through into the inguinal canal.

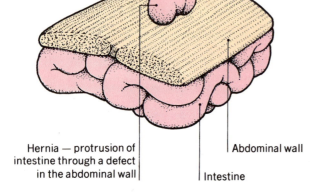

Hernia — protrusion of intestine through a defect in the abdominal wall

Abdominal wall

Intestine

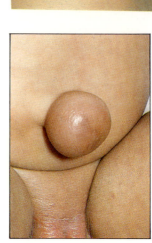

An umbilical hernia may occur when there is a split in the muscles of the abdomen after the stump of the umbilical cord has come away (see left). This is common in babies and almost always disappears without treatment by the time the child is five years old.

Inguinal hernias

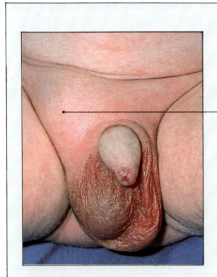

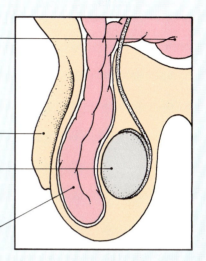

Abdominal cavity

Swelling caused
by inguinal hernia

Penis

Testicle

Loop of intestine coming
down into scrotum

During foetal life the testicle descends from the abdominal cavity into the scrotum through the inguinal canal. The canal largely closes up, but still carries the testicular artery and vein, and the vas deferens which carries the sperms.
In some children the inguinal canal remains open and a loop of intestine can enter into it. This either shows as a lump in the groin (left) or goes right into the scrotum (right). Because of the risk of strangulation of the intestine, inguinal hernias need to be surgically repaired in children.

nia can sometimes get caught so that it does not slip back into place. When this happens the hernia is irreducible and it may give rise to pain and distress. Furthermore, the part of the intestine which is stuck in the hernia may have its blood supply impeded by compression in the canal — doctors refer to this condition as a strangulated hernia. This is a medical emergency.

In children a simple operation can rectify an inguinal hernia. The surgeon pushes the intestine back into the abdominal cavity and stitches the inguinal canal together to close the hole. Sometimes the operation is complicated if the hernia is strangulated. To avoid the risk of strangulation, inguinal hernias in children are repaired as soon as practicable, providing the baby or child is otherwise in good health.

Umbilical hernia

Hernias of the umbilicus (belly button) are extremely common in young children. They appear as a swelling of the umbilicus most noticeable when the baby cries. It is important to realize that the swelling becomes large and tense because the baby is crying, and *not* that the baby is crying because of the swelling.

No treatment is needed for an umbilical hernia in a baby; it gradually gets better during the first year or two, as the gap between the abdominal wall muscles becomes smaller. An umbilical hernia only needs surgical repair if it develops later in life.

Treatment of hernias

Inguinal hernia
To avoid the risk of strangulation, when the part of the intestine stuck in the hernia has its blood supply impeded, inguinal hernais in children are repaired as soon as it is practicable once they have been diagnosed.

Under an anaesthetic the surgeon makes an incision in the groin of the inguinal canal. The intestine is pushed back into the abdominal cavity and the inguinal canal is then stitched together so that the hernia cannot recur. The skin incision is then stitched together. Recovery from the operation is rapid and recurrence of the hernia is rare.

Umbilical hernia
Umbilical hernias are common especially in babies of African descent. They never become irreducible or strangulated so there is no indication for an operation. The defect in the abdominal wall gradually closes and by the age of two almost all umbilical hernias have got better spontaneously.

The urinary system

THE URINARY SYSTEM consists of the kidneys, the ureters, the bladder and the urethra. The kidneys are situated at the back of the abdomen, one on each side of the lumbar spine, and they manufacture urine by removing excess fluid and waste products from the blood stream by selective filtration. From the kidneys the urine flows down the ureters into the bladder. The bladder is a hollow muscular organ which expands as it fills with urine, and then empties by contraction to expel the urine through the urethra to the outside of the body. Emptying of the bladder when it becomes full is an automatic reflex in the first year of life, but it gradually comes under voluntary control as the child develops.

Serious congenital abnormalities of the kidneys are fortunately rare. Sometimes there is total failure of kidney development and the baby dies in the newborn period. Occasionally one or both kidneys are small and poorly developed; this varies in severity depending on the extent. Defective development of the urethra in boys is not uncommon, with the opening being not at the tip of the penis but along the shaft. This is called *hypospadias*.

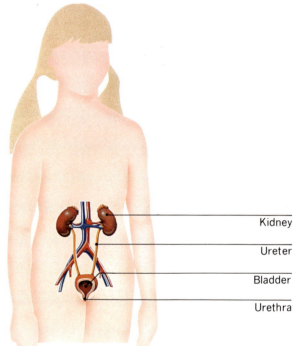

The kidneys filter the blood to remove waste and excess fluid, which is then excreted as urine.

The ureter which carries the urine from the kidney to the bladder.

The bladder acts as a reservoir for urine. It has a muscular wall which, when it contracts, forces the urine through the urethra and enables the bladder to empty completely.

The urethra connects the bladder to the outside.

Kidney

Ureter

Bladder

Urethra

Boys Kidneys are situated at the back of the abdomen, one on each side of the spine. The ureters leading from them carry urine to the bladder. The bladder lies in the pelvis behind the pubic bone. In boys the urethra is long, running from the bladder to the tip of the penis. At the tip of the penis there is an opening which provides an outlet for semen as well as for urine. Hypospaidas is a developmental abnormality in which the urethra opens under the shaft of the penis.

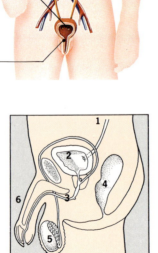

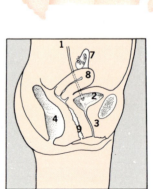

The two illustrations above show cross-sections of a boy and a girl's urinary system and genitalia. Ureter (1), bladder (2), urethra (3), rectum (4), testicle (5), penis (6), ovary (7), uterus or womb (8), vagina (9).

Girls The ureters leading from the kidneys carry urine to the bladder. In girls the urethra is very short, connecting the bladder with the urethral opening at the front of the vulva.

How the kidney works

The kidneys are provided with a large supply of blood via the renal arteries. Their function is to remove waste products and excess fluid from the bloodstream, and to produce urine. Within the kidney the renal artery splits up into branches so that the blood is dispersed throughout the kidney substance.

Within the cortex, or outer layer of the kidney, there are large numbers of glomeruli, each of microscopic size, which consist of a small cluster of blood vessel capillaries at the end of a nephron.

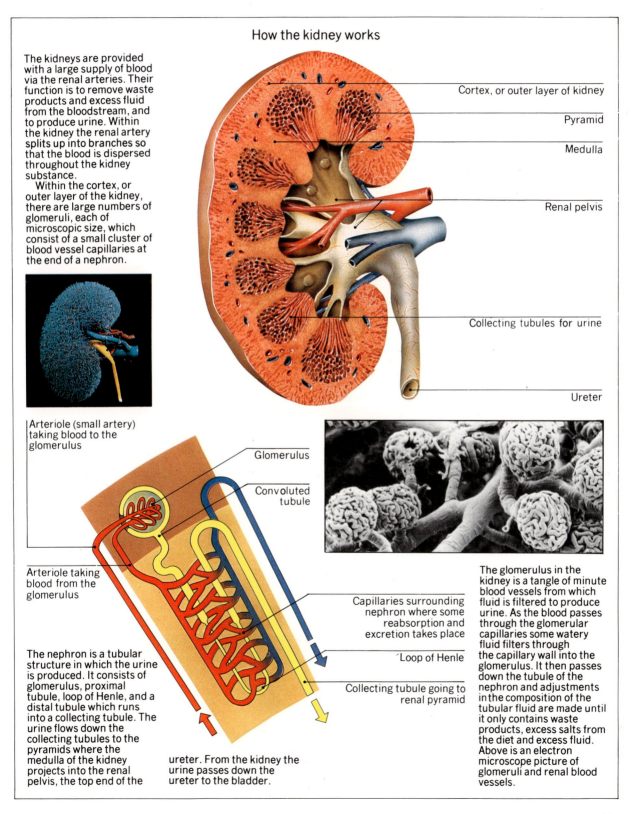

Cortex, or outer layer of kidney

Pyramid

Medulla

Renal pelvis

Collecting tubules for urine

Ureter

Arteriole (small artery) taking blood to the glomerulus

Glomerulus

Convoluted tubule

Arteriole taking blood from the glomerulus

Capillaries surrounding nephron where some reabsorption and excretion takes place

Loop of Henle

Collecting tubule going to renal pyramid

The nephron is a tubular structure in which the urine is produced. It consists of glomerulus, proximal tubule, loop of Henle, and a distal tubule which runs into a collecting tubule. The urine flows down the collecting tubules to the pyramids where the medulla of the kidney projects into the renal pelvis, the top end of the ureter. From the kidney the urine passes down the ureter to the bladder.

The glomerulus in the kidney is a tangle of minute blood vessels from which fluid is filtered to produce urine. As the blood passes through the glomerular capillaries some watery fluid filters through the capillary wall into the glomerulus. It then passes down the tubule of the nephron and adjustments in the composition of the tubular fluid are made until it only contains waste products, excess salts from the diet and excess fluid. Above is an electron microscope picture of glomeruli and renal blood vessels.

Urinary tract infection

INFECTION OF THE URINARY tract is common at all ages. In the newborn period both sexes are equally affected, but thereafter females are much more prone to develop urinary infection than males. The bacteria which cause urinary infections normally live harmlessly in the bowel. If these bacteria overcome the body's natural defences they can get into the urinary tract from below and pass up the urethra into the bladder. This gives rise to infection, known as cystitis, and the bacteria may then spread further up the urinary tract to affect the kidneys. Occasionally the urinary tract becomes infected with bacteria carried from the bowel by the bloodstream.

When a child develops a urinary tract infection, the doctor will want to know which bacterial organism is causing the infection, and will give appropriate therapy, but he will also be interested in whether there is any underlying reason why the natural defences of the body did not give sufficient protection against infection.

In the newborn period reluctance to feed accompanied by general listlessness in a previously well baby may signal the onset of urinary tract infection. There may possibly be a raised temperature but there are seldom any specific signs of either infection or urinary tract involvement. Whenever a baby appears off-colour in this way he should be examined for possible infection. This will include sending urine to the laboratory for bacterial culture, and the investigation will detect a urinary tract infection if one is present.

In older children the features of urinary tract infection are very variable. The infection may come on acutely or may start so gradually that the onset is not noticed.

Symptoms which may be present include fever, malaise, abdominal pain and backache, as well as frequency of urination and pain on passing water, but often only one or two of these symptoms are present and in small children they are sometimes absent altogether.

If the infection starts suddenly the child may have a high fever. The temperature can rise to 41°C/105°F and may be accompanied by rigors, which are attacks of shivering, often violent, associated with fever. Poor appetite, nausea, vomiting and sometimes diarrhoea and blood in the urine are all common in severe acute urinary tract infection. If the onset of infection is more gradual, symptoms may be mainly non-specific, including poor appetite and general malaise. There may be pain on passing water or abdominal pain just after urination, but these are not always present. A frequent desire to pass urine is usual, and in a child who had become dry at nights, bed-wetting may be a feature.

The doctor will want to fully examine a child with these symptoms, and if urinary infection is suspected he will be particularly interested in whether the kidneys are tender or enlarged, and whether or not the bladder is distended. A clean specimen of urine needs to be sent to the laboratory, where they will look and see if there are any inflammatory cells, and culture the sample to see if there is any bacteria present.

If the child is acutely ill the doctor may start treatment with an antibiotic before the urine culture result is available, but often the result is awaited before starting treatment, so that the most suitable anti-bacterial drug can be chosen. As well as giving an antibiotic the

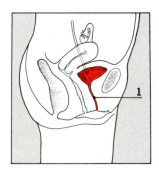

Girls are much more prone to develop urinary infections than boys. The bacteria that cause urinary infections are normal inhabitants of the bowel and the skin of the perineum. On occasion some of them may overcome the body's defences and pass up the urethra into the bladder to cause infection in this area. Because the urethra is short in girls (1), infection spreads up more readily than it does in boys (2), where the urethra is much longer.

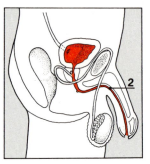

Treatment of urinary infection

When a child has a urinary infection it is important to know which bacteria are causing the infection, and to know which antibiotics the infection will respond to. For this purpose at least one, and preferably two urine specimens should be collected into a clean container and sent to the laboratory.

In the laboratory the specimen is looked at under the microscope and the sample is cultured to grow any bacteria. In this way the most appropriate antibiotic for the particular infection present can be selected. Treatment with an antibiotic will rapidly suppress a urinary infection. A plentiful fluid intake also helps by washing out some of the bacteria every time the bladder is emptied.

After the infection has been treated it is important that follow-up urine specimens go to the laboratory to ensure that the infection has been eradicated. Ideally follow-up should be for several months with occasional urine tests.

The doctor may also want to arrange for Xrays of the urinary tract, such as an IVP and micturating cystogram, and may also want ultrasound pictures of the kidney.

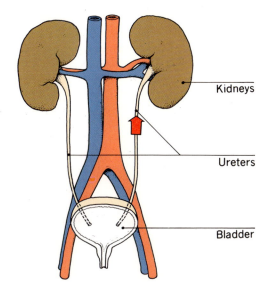

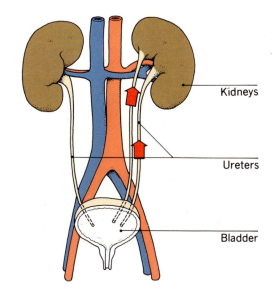

Normally the valves that connect the ureters to the bladder prevent urine from flowing upwards. If the valves do not close properly there is a backflow of urine up the ureter when the bladder empties; this predisposes to infection which can spread upwards and damage the kidney.

A double or duplex ureter is quite a common congenital abnormality. The flow of urine is reduced, being divided into two, and this predisposes to urinary infection. The red arrows indicate the spread of infection. This is highest where urine flows most slowly — in the inside double ureter.

doctor will suggest a plentiful fluid intake. The bacteria grow and increase in numbers in the urine, and passing a large volume of urine frequently helps to rid the bladder of bacteria at a faster rate than they can multiply.

A week or ten days treatment may be sufficient to alleviate the infection, but if it does not settle in this time, or there is a later recurrence, more prolonged treatment may be needed.

When a urinary culture confirms that a child has a urinary infection, and after treatment has been established, the doctor may request a further investigation of the kidneys and urinary system. Most commonly performed are special Xrays. Intravenous pyleography (IVP) consists of a series of films taken at intervals after the injection of a special dye into a vein. The dye is excreted by the kidneys and concentrated in the urine, and the films show details of the kidney, ureters and bladder. Any structural abnormality or obstruction will be identified, and a decision can be made on whether further treatment is warranted.

The micturating cystogram is a series of Xray films taken after a dye has been instilled in the bladder via a CATHETER. By taking pictures as the bladder empties during urination it is possible to see if there is any reflux (backflow) up into the ureters, or any obstruction or urinary outflow. Both reflux and urinary obstruction predispose to recurrent urinary infection, and may require surgical correction if present.

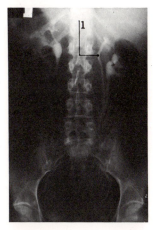

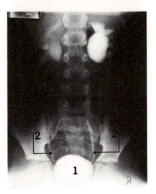

Intravenous pyelography (or urography) known as an IVP (or IVU) is a special Xray to show the kidneys and urinary system. A special dye is injected into a vein and is rapidly concentrated in the kidney, to be excreted in the urine. Because the dye is opaque to Xrays, pictures taken in the hour after the injection show up the urinary tract.

This IVP (see left) shows a congenital anomaly with a double (duplex) ureter on the right side (see 1). This anomaly may be insignificant but sometimes predisposes to urinary infection.

A micturating cystogram is a series of Xray films taken after a dye has been instilled in the bladder. The Xray (see left) is taken while the child is urinating and shows dye both in the bladder (1) and refluxing up the ureters (2).

Genitalia

ANOMALIES OF THE GENITALIA may occur during development and be apparent in childhood. Other diseases of the genitalia are uncommon before puberty.

In girls, because the ovaries and the genitalia are all inside, developmental anomalies are not often apparent in childhood. Minor abnormalities of the womb (uterus) are common, but are seldom detected in childhood. As they are not usually of any medical consequence this is immaterial.

In the few years before puberty it is common for girls to have a slight clear or whitish vaginal discharge and this is no cause for concern. If a girl of any age has a discharge which is excessive, irritant or offensive it may signify an infection (for further details, see vaginal discharge in the glossary).

In boys the testicles and genitalia can be easily examined. Various developmental anomalies occur, and the more common are described below.

Hypospadias

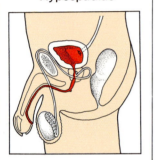

Normally in boys the urethra opens on the tip of the penis. Sometimes the opening is on the underside of the penis (see diagram). This is known as hypospadias. Minor degrees of hypospadias, where the urethra opens near the tip of the penis may not require any treatment, but if the opening is further down the shaft surgical correction may be necessary. In the most severe form of hypospadias the urethra opens on the perineum.

A hydrocoele is a painless fluid-filled cyst in the protective layers around the testis and spermatic cord. It causes swelling in the scrotum, but the testis itself is not involved. If present at birth or soon after, the fluid disappears during infancy without treatment. If it first appears at two or three years, and enlarges during the day and diminishes during the night, spontaneous resolution is rare and surgery will be necessary.

Small intestine	
Spermatic cord	
Penis	
Testis	
Fluid-filled cyst	

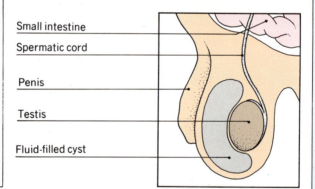

Circumcision

Circumcision for religious or cultural reasons is widely practised. There are seldom any medical reasons for circumcision and it must be remembered that the foreskin has an important protective function as the tip of the penis (the glans) is sensitive and delicate. Unless done for medical reasons the operation should be done only in the first week or two of life when a simple surgical device can be used.

The medical indications for circumcision are repeated ballooning of the foreskin when urine is passed and repeated infections under the foreskin. The operation of circumcision is simple, but complications including infection and haemorrhage can occur. There is discomfort following the operation, and the penis may become inflamed, bruised and swollen. Fortunately healing is normally rapid.

Circumcision must not be performed if *hypospadias* is present, because the tissue of the foreskin may be needed in the future for reconstructive surgery.

Undescended testicle During foetal development the testicles, which originate in the abdominal cavity, migrate downwards into the scrotum (right). At birth they are normally in the scrotum, but in pre-term infants testicular descent may be incomplete.

Sometimes one or both testicles do not descend fully, usually because the testicle gets stuck in the inguinal canal.

An undescended testicle will require an operation in the early childhood years to get it into the right place. Normal pubertal development of the testicle can only take place in the scrotum.

Kidney	
Position of undescended testicle	
Ureters	
Bladder	
Urethra	
Testis	

Bed-wetting

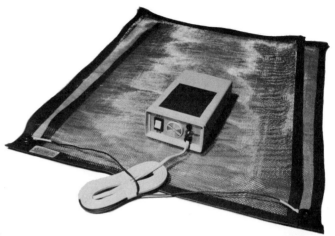

BLADDER CONTROL IS ACQUIRED gradually by a combination of developmental maturation and superimposed learning. In infancy the bladder empties by reflex whenever it is full. Most children have daytime control (barring occasional accidents) by the age of two years, and go on to become dry at nights over the next year or two. By four years the majority of children can go through the night without being wet; about ten per cent of children are still wetting the bed at five years, and about five per cent are not realiably dry by the age of ten

Bed-wetting beyond the age of five years is abnormal, and is referred to as enuresis. Enuresis is more common in boys than girls, and sometimes seems to be familial. It is often unclear why a particular child fails to acquire bladder control. In only a few cases is there an underlying physical problem, such as urinary tract infection. In the majority of children there is no physical cause for the enuresis, and the condition is thought to be emotional.

Major emotional events, such as moving house, birth of a sibling, or family separation, occuring at a time when the child should be acquiring night-time bladder control (around the age of three years) may inhibit the development of that control. If not acquired at the appropriate time, control is harder to achieve later, even though the event provoking it may have been resolved.

Some children who are emotionally insecure or anxious, may have difficulty in becoming dry at night. For some children apprehension about wetting the bed can provoke a vicious circle by inhibiting them from learning control.

Whatever the cause of enuresis the effects are readily apparent. The child becomes ashamed and embarrassed about the problem, although he may attempt an air of unconcern. For the parents there is a continuing worry at the persistence of the symptoms, but training should be based on encouragement; anger at the child will only make matters worse.

Help for enuresis

Many families never seek medical advice about bed-wetting, but if it persists beyond the age of five or six years, it is certainly worth consulting your doctor, or health clinic. The doctor will want to take a history to find out details of the problem, including the current pattern of bed-wetting, the age at which daytime control was achieved, and whether or not there are any other medical or social problems. He will also want to know if the family are trying to do anything to help with the problem, such as restricting drinking in the evening or waking the child to pass urine during the night. The doctor will examine the child and may arrange for a urine specimen to go to the laboratory in order to exclude any infection.

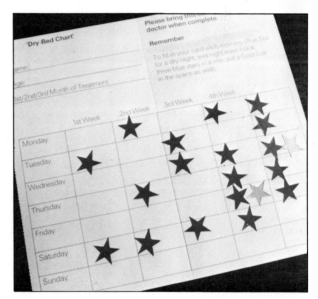

Treatment for enuresis is designed to help the child acquire the skill of nocturnal bladder control. Most widely used are star charts (see above) and enuresis alarms (top) **A star chart** provides a means of involving the child and making him more aware of his problem. Each morning the child has to indicate on the chart whether or not he has woken up with a dry bed. Sticking on stars for dry nights is the usual way of recording. It is important that the child keeps his own chart, and periodically has to show it to the doctor or other therapist to show how he is getting on. The charts provide symbolic recognition of success. By this simple method many children acquire control over a couple of months as the problem is taken outside the family. The **enuresis alarm** is a buzzer that goes off whenever the child wets the bed. Providing the child is woken up by the alarm he will stop night-time wetting within a few days or weeks. The alarm itself consists of a battery and electric buzzer connected to two metal gauze or perforated foil mats which are put into the bed. A dry sheet separates the mats and prevents contact between them. When urine wets the sheet it completes the circuit and sets off the buzzer. Although simple enough in concept, the enuresis alarm requires attention to detail in setting up and parents will need to remake the bed and reset the alarm in the night whenever it goes off. However this effort is soon rewarded as the success rate is high.

The brain and nervous system

THE NERVOUS SYSTEM consists of the brain, the spinal cord, and the nerves. The brain coordinates and controls many of the functions and actions of the body, while the nerves carry impulses to and from the brain to all parts of the body. As such they form the body's communications network.

The main parts of the brain are the right and left cerebral hemispheres, the cerebellum, and the brain stem. The brain inside the skull is well protected from injury, being surrounded by bone, supported by membranes called meninges, and cushioned by a thin layer of fluid (the cerebro-spinal fluid) between the brain and the inside of the skull.

The surface of the cerebral hemisphere is convoluted, which gives it a large surface area. The outer layer, or cortex, contains billions of nerve cells which perform the many and varied cerebral functions. Visual, auditory, and other sensory input data coming to the

brain via the nerves, are analyzed and interpreted by the cerebral cortex. The cortex also initiates and controls body movements, with the left cerebral hemisphere mainly serving the right side of the body, and vice versa. When a person is right-handed the left hemisphere is said to be dominant. Language, learning, thought and intellect are all cerebral functions, and they are mainly located in the dominant hemisphere. Inside each cerebral hemisphere there is a fluid-filled cavity, called the lateral ventricle, which connects with a canal running the whole length of the brain stem and spinal cord. Cerebro-spinal fluid (CSF) circulates through the lateral ventricles and canal system, and around the outside of the brain and spinal cord. HYDROCEPHALUS (water on the brain) may be caused by obstruction to the flow of CSF.

The cerebellum is situated at the back of the brain underneath the cerebral hemispheres. It is concerned

The brain is a highly complex organ as befits its many varied functions. There are various different parts of the brain (see diagram) including the cerebral hemispheres, the cerebellum and the brain stem.

The brain receives nerve impulses from all over the body concerning the different sensations of touch, pressure, position, pain, smell, taste, balance, vision and hearing. The special sense organs, the ears, eyes and nose have nerves which go straight to the brain, whereas the impulses from the rest of the body go from nerves to the spinal cord and then up the brain stem.

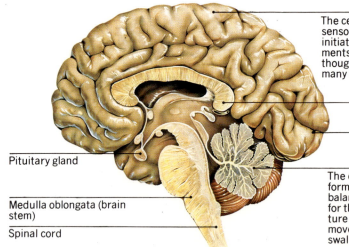

The cerebrum receives sensory information and initiates voluntary movements. It also controls thoughts and speech and has many other functions.

Corpus callosum

Visual area of cortex

The cerebellum receives information on position and balance and is responsible for the maintenance of posture and the coordination of movements, including swallowing and speaking.

Pituitary gland

Medulla oblongata (brain stem)

Spinal cord

Handedness Between the ages of two and three children start to show hand preference, and this continues through life. About 90 per cent of individuals are right-handed and in them the left cerebral hemisphere becomes dominant, not only controlling the movements of the preferred side, but also controlling the use of language and speech. Brain damage to the dominant hemisphere in an adult (such as from a stroke), or in older children, leads to problems both with movement and speech. Brain damage

localized to one hemisphere in infancy leads to the other hemisphere becoming dominant, so that language development can be normal.

Key
1.2.3. Frontal lobes influence behaviour and emotions
4. Speech area
5. Motor cortex
6. Sensory cortex
7. Hearing centre
8. Control of position and posture
9.10 Development of language areas
11. Visual cortex

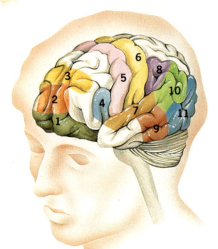

The nerve network

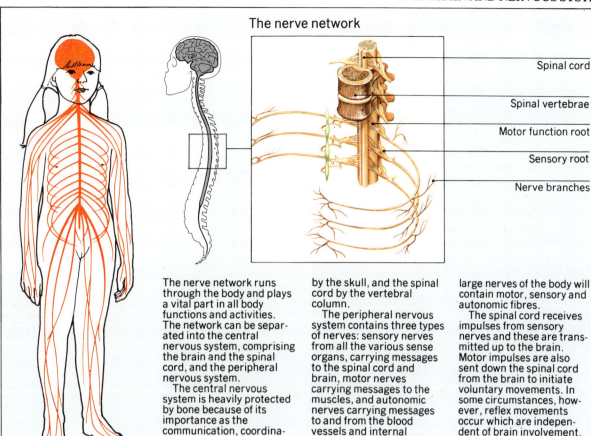

Spinal cord

Spinal vertebrae

Motor function root

Sensory root

Nerve branches

The nerve network runs through the body and plays a vital part in all body functions and activities. The network can be separated into the central nervous system, comprising the brain and the spinal cord, and the peripheral nervous system.

The central nervous system is heavily protected by bone because of its importance as the communication, coordination and intellectual centre of the individual. The brain is encased and supported by the skull, and the spinal cord by the vertebral column.

The peripheral nervous system contains three types of nerves: sensory nerves from all the various sense organs, carrying messages to the spinal cord and brain, motor nerves carrying messages to the muscles, and autonomic nerves carrying messages to and from the blood vessels and internal organs. Often these different types of nerves will all run together, so that the large nerves of the body will contain motor, sensory and autonomic fibres.

The spinal cord receives impulses from sensory nerves and these are transmitted up to the brain. Motor impulses are also sent down the spinal cord from the brain to initiate voluntary movements. In some circumstances, however, reflex movements occur which are independent of brain involvement. Withdrawing from a painful stimulus such as a prick or burn is a reflex action.

Movement and senses

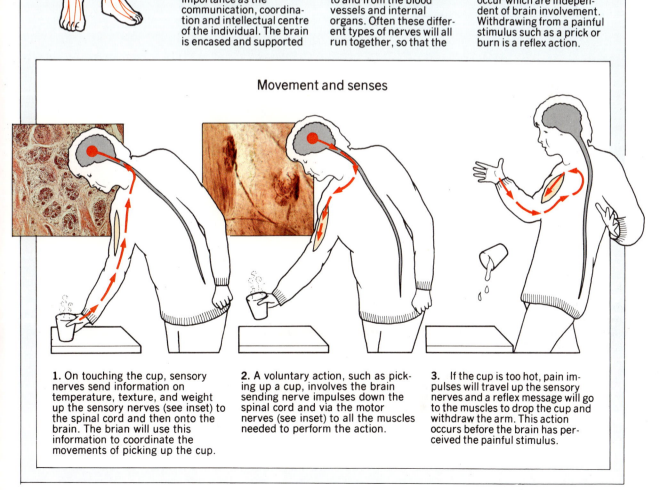

1. On touching the cup, sensory nerves send information on temperature, texture, and weight up the sensory nerves (see inset) to the spinal cord and then onto the brain. The brian will use this information to coordinate the movements of picking up the cup.

2. A voluntary action, such as picking up a cup, involves the brain sending nerve impulses down the spinal cord and via the motor nerves (see inset) to all the muscles needed to perform the action.

3. If the cup is too hot, pain impulses will travel up the sensory nerves and a reflex message will go to the muscles to drop the cup and withdraw the arm. This action occurs before the brain has perceived the painful stimulus.

with balance and with coordinating muscular movements so that they occur in a smooth and controlled manner. This is important for posture, for control of speech and eye movements, as well as for voluntary movement.

The brain-stem connects the cerebral hemispheres to other parts of the brain and to the spinal cord. It carries nerve fibres connecting the cerebral cortex with the rest of the body, and also contains groups of nerve cells called muscle which control vital body functions like sleeping and waking, appetite and digestion, respiration, circulation and body temperature.

The spinal cord is the downward continuation of the brain-stem. The cord runs almost the whole length of the vertebral column (spine) and is protected by a bony arch at the back of each vertebra. The spinal cord is a bundle of thousands of nerve fibres going to and fro from the brain, and pairs of nerves branch from the cord to right and left in each of the gaps between the vertebrae which make up the vertebral column.

The brain and spinal cord are known as the central nervous system, often abbreviated to CNS. The nerves which run from the spinal cord to all the parts of the body comprise the peripheral nervous system. Peripheral nerves are made up of many different nerve fibres, each of which convey nerve impulses and have a specific function. Sensory nerves convey signals of sensation such as touch, position, temperature and pain to the brain from nerve endings in the skin and internal organs. Motor nerves convey stimuli from the brain to the muscles and so initiate movement. Autonomic nerves conduct impulses to control such reflex things as heart rate, blood pressure and digestion.

How doctors examine the nervous system

There are so many different functions of the nervous system that for any one child a medical examination will probably concentrate on only some of the functions. In small children a large amount of information can be obtained from watching the child at play, rather than trying to carry out a series of tests demanding the cooperation of the child. Abnormalities of posture, restriction in spontaneous movement, poor balance or coordination, or developmental delay, may all point to neurological abnormality. Detailed examination of the nervous system may include the following:

Measurement of head size. This gives a check on brain growth and will detect *hydrocephalus* (water on the brain), if this is present.

Looking for neck stiffness. Neck movements are restricted in meningitis and sometimes in cerebral irritation. Bending the head forward causes pain, or movement is limited.

Looking into the eyes. The optic nerve, and the retina

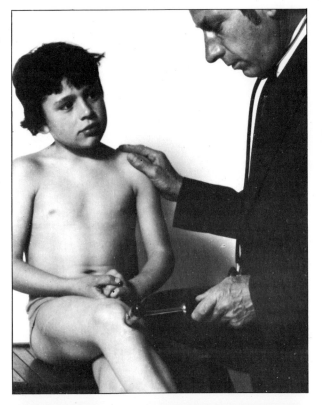

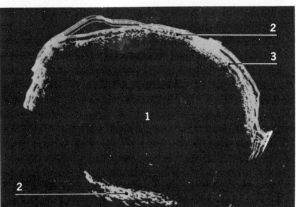

Testing reflexes (top)When the doctor tests the reflexes with a rubber hammer he is checking both sensory and motor pathways.

If either sensory or motor nerve is non-functional there will be no reflex jerk. If the sensory and motor nerves are intact, but there is damage to the motor nerves in the brain or spinal cord, the reflex will be exaggerated.

Ultrasound can be used to identify internal bleeding in babies after birth, and to show the size of the ventricles (brain cavities containing fluid).

Above is an ultrasound view of the head (facing right) in a baby with hydrocephalus. There is enormous dilatation of the ventricles (shown black, 1). The white surround consists of bone (2) and cerebral cortex (3) which is thinner than normal.

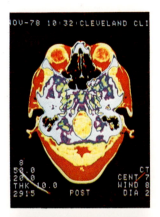

Computerized tomography is a special Xray technique. By rotating an Xray beam around the head, measuring the image in many different positions and computer analysing the results, it is possible to obtain detailed information about the structures inside the head. The illustration (top left) shows a computerized tomography picture of a normal child which appears like a cross-section of the head, showing the skull, eyes, cerebrum, cerebellum and brain stem.

Nuclear magnetic resonance is a new technique which gives another way of visualizing the inside of the head. This diagram (left) shows a blood clot (1) on the brain.

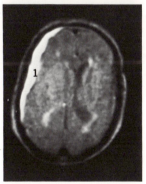

Lumbar puncture

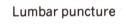

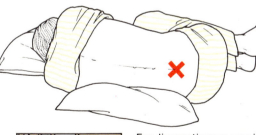

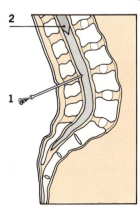

For diagnostic purposes it may be necessary to obtain a sample of the cerebral spinal fluid (CSF). A needle (1) is inserted between two lumbar vertebrae into the fluid-filled space. As the spinal cord (2) ends above the site of the needle insertion, it cannot be damaged by the procedure. The patient lies down, curled up, and the needle is directed between two of the vertebrae, as shown in the diagrams. This investigation is done under local anaesthetic.

and its blood vessels can be seen directly with an opthalmoscope.

Checking movements. The cranial nerves coming from the brain-stem control the movements of the eyes, face, mouth, tongue, and palate. These are each checked in turn. Any abnormality gives a clue to the site and type of any neurological movements.

Motor power and coordination. The strength of the different muscle groups in the arms and legs is tested by getting the child to flex and extend the elbows and knees, wrists and ankles, with the examiner resisting the movement. Coordination can be assessed by watching the child perform rapid movements. Observing the child's posture, way of standing and walking will help in the assessment.

Sensation. The sensation in the skin can be tested using a finger, or cottonwool to assess light touch, and sometimes reaction to a pin prick is tried. Absent sensation over an area of skin suggests malfunction of the sensory nerves.

Reflexes. Normally a muscle contraction can be induced by banging the muscle tendon with a rubber hammer. The doctor may look for elbow, knee and ankle jerks in this way. In spastic children the jerks are exaggerated; where there is nerve damage or muscular dystrophy the jerks are reduced.

Testing vision and hearing. Visual and auditory problems sometimes have a neurological cause. It is very important that they are properly tested in a child who has other evidence of brain damage.

Lumbar puncture (L.P). In suspected meningitis and some other neurological conditions it is necessary to obtain a sample of cerebro-spinal fluid (CSF) for laboratory testing. The spinal cord ends in the lumbar region (lower back) while the membranes surrounding the cord extend further down. A fine needle is inserted between the lumbar vertebrae to obtain a sample.

Xrays. Xrays of the skull will occasionally give useful information about the brain. Nerve tissue which is soft does not show up on normal Xrays and more information can be obtained from a brain scan.

Brain scan. Pictures of the structures inside the head can be obtained using a technique called computerized tomography (CT). A special Xray machine linked to a computer swings round the head and produces detailed pictures of the brain structure. It can detect lesions within or around the brain.

Ultrasound. Ultrasound can be used to visualize internal structures, and is useful for studying the heads of babies. In the newborn it can detect internal bleeding, and in infants it can be used to test for early HYDROCEPHALUS.

Electroencephalogram (EEG). A record of the electrical activity of the brain (see page 119).

Faints and convulsions

SUDDEN LOSS OF CONSCIOUSNESS in a child may be due to a convulsion, a breath-holding attack, or a faint.

Convulsions. A convulsion, seizure or fit is a disturbance of the brain function which in children could be due to epilepsy or to a raised body temperature. Less commonly, fits may be caused by other conditions such as meningitis, very low blood pressure, or poisoning with certain anti-depressant drugs. In a major seizure, as well as sudden loss of consciousness, there may be stiffness of the body, followed by jerking of the limbs. Other forms of seizure are mentioned later under *epilepsy*.

Faints. A faint is an episode of loss of consciousness due to a temporary reduction in the supply of blood going to the brain. Fainting is more common in adolescence than in early childhood, and may occur with prolonged standing, particularly if it is hot and stuffy, or because of a sudden emotional shock. As soon as the child loses consciousness and falls down the blood supply to the brain improves, and recovery is rapid. *For first aid treatment of convulsions and faints, see page 181.*

Breath-holding spells. Toddlers, when they are hurt or cross, may hold their breath for a few seconds before letting out a cry. In some children the breath-holding is more prolonged and they pass out. As soon as they lose consciousness normal breathing resumes, and within a minute or two recovery is complete.

Febrile convulsions

Some children under the age of five years develop a convulsion if they get a raised temperature. The parents may have been aware earlier that the child is unwell, but as the convulsions occur most commonly as the temperature is going up at the start of the illness, they can occur without any warning.

Most parents are very frightened at seeing a fit, as the child suddenly loses consciousness and starts to twitch and go blue in the face. Fortunately febrile convulsions are usually short, lasting only a few minutes. During the convulsions the child should be turned onto his side on the bed or floor, with the face turned downwards so that any moisture in the mouth will drain out. Nothing should be forced between the teeth or gums, neither should the child be wrapped up, as this will raise the temperature even further.

If a child has had a fit, medical advice should be sought, and most children are admitted to hospital for observation and investigation with their first febrile convulsion. If the convulsion goes on for more than five minutes medical help should be sought urgently. If the child is still convulsing when seen by the doctor, he will probably give an injection to stop the fit, and institute measures which will help to lower the temperature of the body, such as removing the clothes and tepid sponging. Once the convulsion is over the medical problem is to discover the cause of the fever, give any necessary treatment and care, and decide whether or not the episode was a simple febrile convulsion, or caused by some other factor.

Further investigations may be necessary, including sometimes a lumbar puncture to make certain that there is no evidence of infection of the nervous system itself.

If your child has lost consciousness or is having a fit, place him in the recovery position with the head back as shown on page 175. This is the correct position for recovery as it is comfortable, makes breathing easier and prevents the tongue from falling to the back of the throat. When you have put the child in this position, stay with him and, if he is having a convulsion, do not restrain him except to make sure he is not injuring himself. Do not put anything into his mouth.

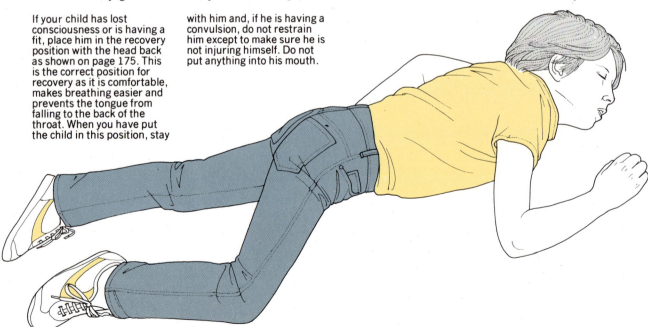

Occasionally the doctor may arrange an EEG test (*see page 119*) after a febrile convulsion, but this is not usually indicated.

Treatment

When a child has had a febrile convulsion there are three aspects to treatment. Firstly, to treat the cause of the fever; secondly, to give symptomatic treatment to lower the temperature, and to lessen the likelihood of further fits during the current illness; thirdly, to consider the possibility of prevention of convulsions in future illnesses. Whether or not a specific treatment is necessary for the underlying cause of the fever will depend on what the cause is. Some infections will warrant antibiotic treatment; others will be expected to subside spontaneously.

Controlling the body temperature is necessary for all children who have had a febrile convulsion, but anticonvulsant drugs are seldom used following a single convulsion.

Control of fever

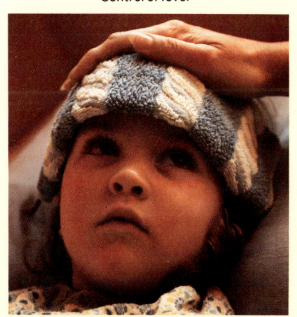

If you realize your child is unwell you should take his temperature, and if this is raised significantly and the child is feverish, follow the measures outlined below. **Remove clothes** A child with a fever should be either naked or in light clothing; thick bedclothes should be avoided. As a child loses heat from the body through the skin it is not possible to reduce his temperature effectively if he is well covered. **Give plenty of fluids** A feverish child will frequently have a poor appetite. Plenty of sweet, cool drinks help to provide energy, prevent dehydration, and may reduce the temperature and make the child more comfortable. **Sponge the child** Lukewarm water over the face and body will also help to lower the temperature. The child should be dried with a towel before the sponging process is repeated. Do not sponge the child for more than half an hour at a time, and the whole process should not be repeated more frequently than every two hours, or the child will lose too much body heat. An electric fan, if available, will also help cooling. **Prevention** A child who has had one febrile convulsion may have another anytime he gets a raised temperature, although half the children affected in this way only ever have one convulsion. The tendency to febrile convulsions will have been outgrown by the age of five.

If a significant rise in temperature can be prevented, this should stop a convulsion from occurring. Sometimes however, the onset of a convulsion is the first indication that the child is unwell.

Anti-convulsant drugs are not given as a matter of course to children who have had one or two febrile convulsions, unless the fits have been particularly severe. If the child has had several episodes, the doctor may consider a period of regular medication to try and prevent further convulsions.

Junior dosage of aspirin and paracetamol

Soluble aspirin or paracetamol will lower a child's temperature. If the temperature is only just above normal (below 99.5°F/38°C) medication is not necessary. If your child's temperature is higher then the following doses may be given.

AGE	SOLUBLE ASPIRIN	or PARACETAMOL ELIXIR (120 mg in 5 ml)
1 - 2 years	1 junior tablet (75 mg)	5 ml of elixir (120 mg)
2 - 3 years	2 junior tablets (150 mg)	5 - 10 ml of elixir (120 - 240 mg)
3 - 5 years	3 junior tables (225 mg)	10 ml of elixir (240 mg)

This dose may be repeated every 6 hours for up to 24 hours. If needed for a longer period the dose may need to be reduced. **Remember** that both aspirin and paracetamol are potentially dangerous, so return the bottle to a safe place after each dose.

Epilepsy

EPILEPSY IS A TENDENCY to have repeated seizures. The interval between each seizure episode is variable; in some there will be several months between attacks, whilst in other children the attacks can occur daily or every few days. Apart from the intermittent seizures, brain function in epilepsy is often otherwise completely normal.

There are a number of underlying problems which can give rise to epilepsy. In some children subject to recurrent fits there will be brain damage with other associated features, such as cerebral palsy, or mental handicap. In a few there may be other neurological diseases, while in many children who have fits no cause can be found, even after investigation. For this last group doctors use the term idiopathic epilepsy, which means epilepsy of unknown cause.

Convulsions occuring in the newborn period, and convulsions associated with fever, even if they are recurrent, are not considered to be due to epilepsy.

There are several different types of epilepsy, classified by the nature of the seizures. Most common are major seizures and absence seizures.

Major seizures (Tonic-clonic, or grand mal seizures)

In a major seizure consciousness is lost suddenly and the child will fall down. There may be no warning, or the child may cry out at the start of the attack. Some mothers recognize a change of mood in their child, which indicates that a seizure is imminent. The loss of consciousness is associated at first with stiffness of all the muscles of the body (the tonic phase) and then by a generalized jerking (the clonic phase) of the body and limbs. During this period the child goes blue in the face as breathing is interrupted by the convulsion, and there may be frothing at the mouth, or the tongue may be bitten. There may be more than one tonic and clonic phase during a seizure. The child will usually pass urine during an attack.

The seizure continues for a variable period, but is usually less than five minutes. At the end of the seizure the child relaxes, normal breathing is resumed, his colour improves, and he wakes. A major seizure is often followed by a severe headache and the child may want to sleep for a while afterwards.

Absence seizures (petit mal seizures)

Absence seizures consist of short attacks of loss of consciousness only lasting a few seconds. The child does not fall, and usually there are no abnormal movements. To the observer the child just looks blank and unresponsive to his surroundings, and he is probably unaware that an attack has occurred. If absence seizures occur very frequently they can interfere with learning in a classroom situation, as the child will not follow all that is going on.

Other types of epilepsy

There are other rare types of epilepsy, with different types of seizures. They include drop attacks (akinetic seizures), myoclonic epilepsy, infantile spasms, and psychomotor or temporal lobe epilepsy.

Treatment

When asking about the illness the doctor will want to have a description of the attacks and to know when and how often they have occurred. In some children the

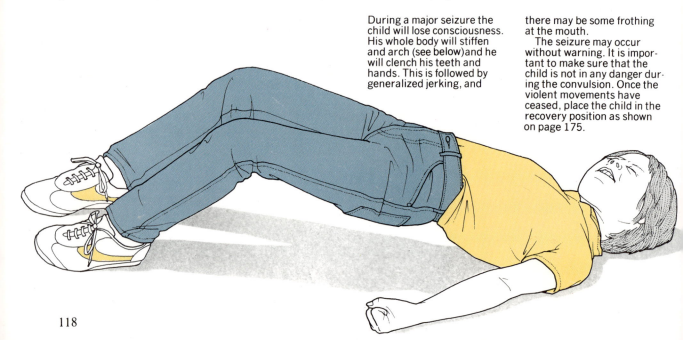

During a major seizure the child will lose consciousness. His whole body will stiffen and arch (see below) and he will clench his teeth and hands. This is followed by generalized jerking, and there may be some frothing at the mouth.

The seizure may occur without warning. It is important to make sure that the child is not in any danger during the convulsion. Once the violent movements have ceased, place the child in the recovery position as shown on page 175.

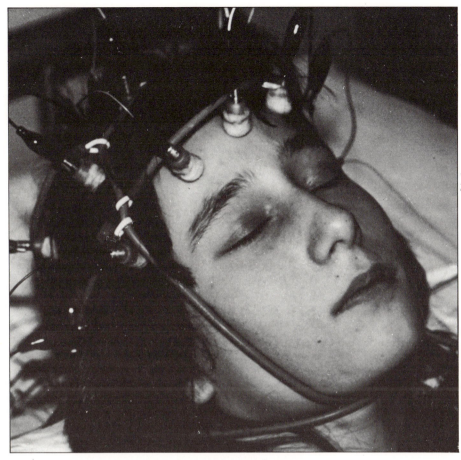

Electroencephalography (EEG) is the method of recording changes of electrical potential in the brain, used in the diagnosis of epilepsy and some other disorders.

Small electrodes are pasted onto the scalp and spaced out to cover the whole of the head. These electrodes are connected to recording pens, and the controls of the machine allow tracings to be made on moving sheets of paper. This written record is called an electroencephalogram

The two diagrams below show examples of tracings given by an EEG during a major seizure and a 'petit mal' seizure.
The left-hand detail records a reading of normal brain activity leading into a major seizure. The right-hand detail shows the characteristic 'spike and wave' trace of the 'petit mal' seizure.

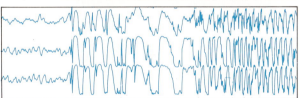

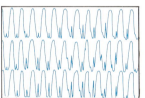

seizures are provoked by flashing lights. Attacks may be precipitated by a malfunctioning fluorescent tube, or by getting too close to a flickering television. The doctor will also want to know about the child's past medical history, general health and development, and any other symptoms. The child will be examined, with particular emphasis on the nervous system. After this the doctor will be able to make a firm diagnosis of epilepsy, but he will also be trying to ascertain if there is any underlying cause.

Further investigations may be necessary. Those most commonly performed are the electroencephalogram (EEG) and a skull Xray. Occasionally the doctor will arrange for a brain scan to help confirm the diagnosis and determine the type of epilepsy. Absence seizures, for instance, can only be confidently diagnosed when the characteristic EEG changes are found.

Epilepsy is treated with anti-convulsant medication with the aim of preventing further seizures. There are several different kinds of medication with anti-convulsant effects, some of which are specially suited to a particular type of epilepsy. The physician starts treatment with one drug selected as likely to be the most

useful, and gradually increases the dose until a level is reached at which seizures are controlled completely without significant side-effects. Regular medication is essential. Forgotten doses and irregular adminstration prevent effective seizure control. Most anti-convulsant drugs are sedative and in large doses can cause drowsiness or unsteadiness. The dose must be carefully adjusted for each individual child. If complete seizure control is not obtained with one drug, an alternative can be added or substituted.

The activities of a child with epilepsy should not necessarily be restricted, but although complete prevention of seizures is the aim, this is not always possible. If occasional seizures persist, it may be necessary to restrain certain activities which could put the child at risk. Unaccompanied swimming, and bicycle riding in traffic are obviously potentially dangerous situations.

Treatment with anti-convulsant drugs is usually continued for two or three years after the last seizure. The drugs are then gradually discontinued to see if they are still necessary. Many children outgrow the tendency to suffer from epilepsy with time, and many are able to discontinue treatment completely.

Mentalhandicap

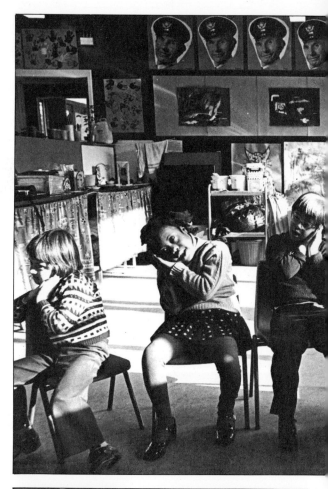

INDIVIDUALS VARY WIDELY in their intelligence. With regard to children, some are very intelligent or bright and are quick to learn new facts and skills, the majority are of average intelligence, and some are dull, being below the average. Children with mental handicap (or mental retardation) have the disability of sub-normal intelligence. Mental handicap is not the same as mental illness, in which there are disturbances of feelings, thoughts or behaviour, but usually normal intelligence.

Mental handicap may be mild, with intellectual ability not far below the normal range, and this actually represents the lower extreme of the normal variation, rather than indicating any underlying disease or brain damage as a cause of the disability.

When mental handicap is more severe, it is due to some form of brain maldevelopment, damage, or malfunction. Any condition causing intellectual impairment may also affect other functions of the brain, and there may be associated disabilities such as *cerebral palsy*, impairment of vision or hearing, or *epilepsy*.

Causes of mental handicap

Mental handicap arises from maldevelopment, damage, or impaired function of the part of the brain which is concerned with intellect. Many different causes are known, and some of the more common are shown in the table.

It is worth trying to find the cause when it is first realized that the child has a handicap. In a few conditions specific treatment is available, as for example, hormone treatment for children with thyroid deficiency, or dietary treatment for PHENYLKETONURIA. Even if no specific therapy is available, if the cause of the handicap is known, it is possible to say whether or not there are any genetic implications, and whether or not there is any chance of a couple having another affected child (*see Genetic counselling, page 45*). Furthermore, if the cause of the handicap is known it may help both in predicting the likely degree of further disability and in coming to terms with the disability itself. If the cause is not apparent, the doctors will investigate to try and determine the cause. These investigations may include chromosome studies and blood and urine tests to measure various body chemical levels, such as thyroid hormone, sugar, calcium, and aminoacids. In some children a brain scan may be done. In spite of investigation, in many children it is not possible to find a cause of mental handicap.

Realizing that a child is mentally handicapped

If the child has characteristic features of a disorder known to be associated with mental handicap, such as Down's syndrome, it may be apparent from birth or early infancy. Often the realization that a child is handi-

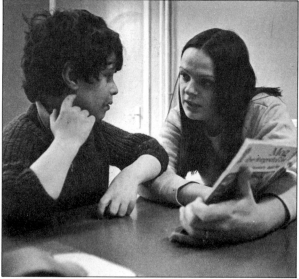

Children with mental handicap need to be assessed early on, firstly to find out whether they suffer from other defects of this condition, such as poor vision and hearing which might be contributing to their educational difficulties, and secondly so that they can be placed in the correct kind of school. A child with a mental handicap is likely to learn more slowly than other children and therefore needs special schooling. For example, a higher staff ratio is needed so that the child can receive plenty of attention and encouragement. Regular assessments should be conducted at intervals to make sure that the child is correctly placed educationally.

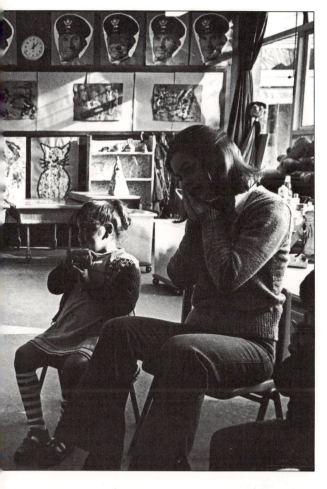

Some causes of mental handicap	
Genetic disorders	Phenylketonuria Tay Sachs disease
Chromosomal disorders	Down's Syndrome (mongolism)
Problems in pregnancy	Intrauterine infections, eg rubella, cytomegalus virus Toxins, eg excess alcohol, some drugs Irradiation with Xrays Nutritional deficiencies
Around the time of birth	Severe oxygen shortage Birth trauma
Newborn period	Severe jaundice Very low blood sugar Thyroid deficiency
After birth	Severe meningitis Severe head injury Lead poisoning

capped comes gradually when there is a delay in achieving normal developmental milestones, such as smiling, gaining head control, sitting, crawling, and starting to talk.

There are, however, wide variations in normal development and other causes of delayed milestones, so a full assessment of the child and his abilities will be needed. Any parent who is worried about a child's development should consult the doctor or child health clinic. To delay seeking help because of anxiety may deprive the child of benefit if treatment is needed. If the child is found to be developing normally, it will relieve parental anxiety.

In infancy or early childhood, it may be impossible for the doctor to decide whether or not there is mental handicap, particularly if it is mild. Even when mental handicap is recognized, it is impossible at first to accurately predict future attainment. Although intellectual ability is partly related to the structure of the brain, it is also considerably influenced by other factors. For all children, adequate nutrition and good physical health, a stable home life, and a stimulating environment with plentiful opportunities for learning, all have a favourable influence on intelligence. They are especially important for children with limited potential.

Care of the mentally handicapped child

Curative treatment is unfortunately only available for a few of the conditions causing mental handicap. For most affected children, the disability has to be accepted, and treatment directed at minimizing the handicap. This treatment is not medical, but consists of seeking to provide those conditions which any child needs for healthy development. There is, however, a need in the early years for continuing medical involvement.

Children with mental handicap often have associated disabilities, including other congenital abnormalities, such as *cerebral palsy*, seizures, and visual or hearing difficulties. They will need regular assessment in early childhood to detect and treat any of these associated abnormalities. They will also need developmental assessments from time to time from a psychologist or a doctor experienced in caring for handicapped children. This assessment will be of use in identifying particular areas that will need special attention, for instance, whether the child would benefit from speech therapy, or should join a nursery group to learn to socialize with his peers. School placement needs to be appropriate, and these assessments will help in this.

In caring for young handicapped children, there needs to be cooperative teamwork between the parents and any professionals involved. Professionals may be able to provide support, guidance and help, but inevitably the main burden of care falls on the parents. Every child and every family is different, and unless there is full discussion between the different people involved in the care, it will not be possible to work out a satisfactory care and management plan for the child. All children need an emotionally secure family background if they are to develop fully and avoid behavioural difficulties. This also applies to children with mental handicap, but inevitably there are unusual stresses and anxieties in a family with a handicapped child, and this can make difficulties for the whole family.

A lot of very important early learning for children comes through play, and the interaction it brings with parents and other people. Because they are slower to learn and to develop social skills than other children, those with mental handicap have a special need of this interaction. The slowness and muted reactions of the child to stimulation do tend to interfere with the parent's enjoyment of the game, and can lead to a reduction in the amount of play with the child.

Therapy

A children's physiotherapist, or occupational therapist experienced in working with small children should be able to help in suggesting different ways the parents can stimulate the child and aid the learning process. The therapist will also be able to advise on which areas of development should be encouraged at a particular time. Children with mental handicap follow a normal pattern of development, but at a slower than normal rate. There is, therefore, no point in trying to encourage standing until balance is good and crawling has been mastered.

Language development is important, and the advice of a speech therapist may be helpful. Both the development of imaginative play, social interaction and communication are needed for language development and the acquisition of speech.

Although a lot of the management of mentally handicapped children concentrates on developing their intellectual abilities to the full, it must be remembered that intellect is only part of personality, and that other aspects of personality are equally, if not more, important. The development of a sense of humour and spirit of fun, the ability to make friends, to enjoy music, to be kind and caring are all things which should be encouraged in the development of children.

The child's handicap may cause increased financial demands on the family, and may even mean that there is less to spend on toys or educational aids. There are, fortunately, a growing number of 'toy libraries' where children can borrow toys that will help in encouraging development. A social worker should be able to make sure the family is getting all the benefits to which they are entitled.

Children with mental handicap are likely to need special schooling, as they will learn more slowly than other children. Regular assessment of intelligence before school starts and at intervals thereafter, will

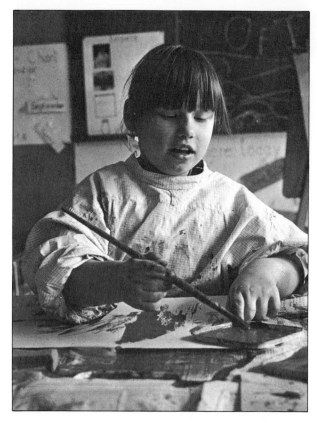

Children with mental handicap have special needs. They are slower to learn than other children and their handicaps can prevent them acquiring social skills which other children pick up easily. This means that they have a special need of interaction and communication with other people so that they can, in their own time, learn to do and enjoy a variety of different things. It is vitally important to play with mentally handicapped children — much is learnt through play. Similarly the environment should be explored and experiences broadened as much as possible as this all helps normal development. The photographs above show mentally handicapped children painting (top left), rowing (top right) and playing in the water (bottom right). These are just a few of the activities that they can participate in and enjoy.

make sure that the child is appropriately placed. Outside of school the child should be encouraged to do as many different and interesting things as possible, to broaden experience. Going on shopping expeditions, which will involve travelling on public transport, can be enjoyable for the child and activities such as swimming, cycling and horse-riding are therapeutic and pleasurable for some handicapped children.

Many children with mild mental handicap grow up to lead completely independent adult lives, with a job and children of their own. With more severe disability, it is likely that sheltered employment and some assistance in organizing their lives will be needed. Society is gradually coming to realize its responsibility in providing ongoing help.

Mental handicap and the family

Having a child with mental handicap poses special problems for the family. These problems include direct results of the handicap, such as having to carry around a

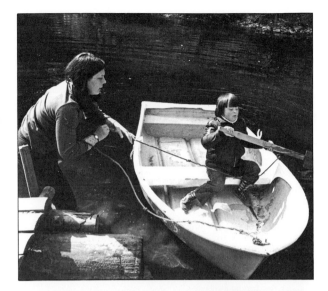

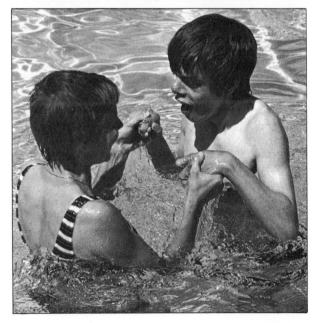

faced, can they be converted into love and care for the child, and a realistic recognition of the disability. Nearly all parents go through a time when they would like to reject the child because of his handicap. Coming to terms with the disability means accepting that you have a child who is an individual to be cherished, but who has special needs that many other children do not have.

It is easier to accept that a child is handicapped if you receive support, explanation, and help in the early weeks after learning of the disability. Some of this support may come from your own doctor, the hospital, or other health care professionals. Much of it will come from the family itself. Additionally, meeting other parents with the same problem may help. Providing the handicapped child with care, appropriate stimulation, and teaching to enable him to make the most of the abilities he does have is a positive way of dealing with the problem. Forever seeking medical opinion in the hope of benefit is one form of non-acceptance which is not in the best interests of the child or the family. When it is first realized that the child is handicapped, many people naturally want a second opinion. Your doctor will cooperate in helping to arrange this, but only in exceptional circumstances will there be a need to obtain further opinions on the problem.

Inevitably, the time taken in caring for a handicapped child, and the associated anxieties, place a continuous strain on the parents and on their marriage. It is necessary for them to find some time to be alone together, and they should not feel guilty about leaving the child with a babysitter, or in a nursery or a children's home while they are on holiday. The strain on the marriage is also relieved if both parents are able to accept the disability and share in providing for the special needs of the child. For some couples this acceptance and sharing deepens and enriches their relationship.

Having a handicapped brother or sister influences the development of other children in the family. They may be deprived of necessary love and encouragement because of parental involvement with the handicapped child, and may resent the attention being given to their sibling. They may also feel a social stigma in having a disabled brother or sister. They should receive understanding and help with these feelings, and it is important that there are times when they can have the undivided attention of their parents. It may help if they are taught, by their parents, to understand the special needs of the handicapped child and encouraged to help in looking after a disabled brother or sister.

The family with a handicapped child is a family with special needs. These needs are not always met by society as well as they should be, but there is an increasing awareness of the problems, and a realization that more should be done to help such families in any way possible.

heavy child who has not yet learned to walk, and needing to spend a lot of time in explaining and assisting with everything, including everyday activities such as feeding, dressing and toiletting. Apart from these problems, there may be difficulties over the need for hospital visits and over setting aside time for therapy or educational play. Perhaps the greatest problem of all for the parents and the rest of the family is to come to terms with the disability, to be able to cope realistically with the handicap, and to be able to face the future with equanimity.

When it is first realized that a child may be mentally handicapped the parents will have very mixed feelings. There will be anxiety and sadness, but also disbelief and a sense of disappointment and loss. There may also be times when there is anger and perhaps guilt and shame. All of these feelings are natural and people who are experienced at working with handicapped families are well aware of them, as are other parents of handicapped children. Only if these feelings can be accepted and

Cerebral palsy

SOME PARTS OF THE brain control the movement and balance of the body. If these areas do not develop properly, or are damaged in early life, either before or after birth, the child will have a problem with muscle control. This physical handicap is known as cerebral palsy.

The most common form of cerebral palsy affects the muscles which become stiff because of overactive contraction. This is known as muscle spasticity, hence the alternative name of spastics for people affected with cerebral palsy. Spastic muscles do not easily perform natural movements, and the overactive contraction may lead to abnormal posture and to deformities of the joints. Not all children with cerebral palsy have stiff spastic muscles. Some are excessively floppy with poor muscle tone and power, and others have difficulty in controlling movements. The different types of cerebral palsy are sometimes mixed.

Cerebral palsy varies greatly in severity. It may be so mild that it only causes a minor problem in one limb, or it may affect the whole body. Many children with the

Cerebral palsy occurs as a result of damage to the developing brain, affecting the areas that control movement. Interruption of the oxygen supply to the brain during birth is a frequent cause of cerebral palsy, but it may also be due to such things as intrauterine infection, or trauma during or after birth.
Damage may not be confined to the motor areas of the brain so there may be associated disability, such as visual impairment or mental handicap.
The disability in cerebral palsy may only affect part of the body. If one half of the body is paralysed (yellow area) it is called **hemiplegia** (top); when only the legs are affected it is known as **diplegia** or **paraplegia** (middle); and if all four limbs are involved it is known as **quadriplegia** (bottom).

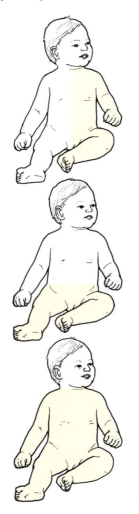

Testing for Handicap

Cerebral palsy may be suspected because of limited movement of a limb on one side of the body. The doctor looks for asymmetry (1) when the baby moves, and feels for either excessive stiffness of the muscles when the limbs are moved (2) or excessive floppiness. Both can indicate nerve damage. Slowness in achieving motor milestones, and abnormal postures and reactions can indicate motor abnormalities. The tendon jerks, tested with a patellar hammer (3), are often brisk in cerebral palsy.

disease have no other associated problems, but if the underlying brain damage affects other areas, apart from those concerned with movement, there may be associated handicaps such as intellectual or visual impairment. The features of cerebral palsy are very variable depending on the type, the parts of the body affected, and the severity. Furthermore, the features may alter as the child grows and develops.

A child with cerebral palsy may not have any obvious abnormality of movements immediately after birth, but gradually as the child grows it may be realized that there are less spontaneous movements than in other children. This may be noticeable if only one limb or one side of the body is affected, because of the contrast with the other side. The stiffness, or spasticity, of the muscles is not often apparent in the early months of life, and in fact, the baby may at first be rather floppy with poor head control.

By the time the child is a few months old it is likely that either the abnormality of movement will have been noted, or slowness in achieving motor milestones will have alerted the parents to seek medical aid. If the

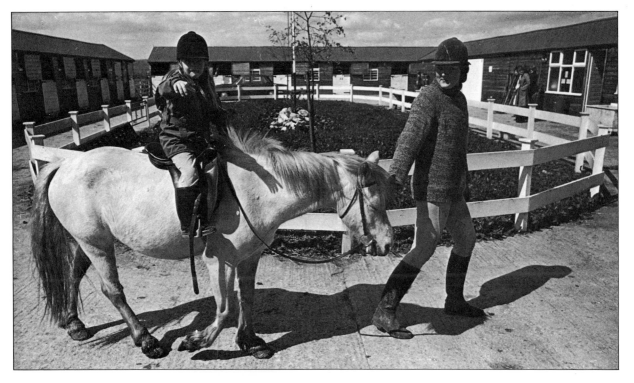

Children with disabilities often become additionally handicapped as they are unable to learn by exploring their environment. Horse riding for the handicapped is a way of providing both physical exercise and broadening the child's outlook, and has proved to be very important therapeutically for many handicapped children.

disability is mild, and particularly if only the legs are affected, it may not be noted until after the child has started to walk.

When the doctor sees a child with suspected movement problems, he will want to observe the child's reaction in responding to being rolled over and pulled up to a sitting position. He will also want to feel the flexibility of the limbs, and test the reflexes, and do a thorough general examination. It may not be possible to be definite about a diagnosis, or even to decide whether or not there is a problem when the child is first seen. It may need repeated examinations over a period of time to fully assess the problem. Special investigations, such as Xrays or blood tests, are seldom indicated in cerebral palsy.

In cerebral palsy treatment is needed to encourage natural movements, to improve balance and control, to foster developmental progress, and to prevent contractures. In addition, the medical, educational, social or emotional needs of the child and the family must be met.

Much of the treatment for the locomotor problem will be under the guidance of a physiotherapist, working both with the child and with the parents, instructing them on suitable positions for the child when lying and sitting, on passive movements to be done daily, and on how to encourage natural movements. Obviously a therapist with experience of working with disabled children is preferable and this may mean the need to attend a special centre for treatment.

The paediatrician will see the child regularly to assess progress, and an orthopaedic surgeon may need to be consulted. Some children with cerebral palsy may require operations to prevent, or correct, deformities which can arise from unequal muscle action, or to free a joint which does not straighten fully.

Inevitably, if a child has a disability, there are extra needs and family stresses. A social worker may be able to help by finding additional financial and caring resources to help the family. Many parents also get support from joining a national or local parents group.

Although cerebral palsy interferes with normal locomotor development, with appropriate management most children steadily improve in ability throughout childhood, and the disability becomes less pronounced.

Headaches

HEADACHES ARE COMMON in childhood. Most are trivial and get better quickly, either spontaneously or after a simple analgesic such as paracetamol or soluble aspirin. These are often associated with tiredness or anxiety and are not of great significance.

Some children get more severe headaches, which may be frequent, and may at times disrupt normal activities. Most commonly these are due to migraine, or to stress, but consideration has to be given to the possibility of other underlying causes for the headaches. The onset of a headache associated with a raised temperature is suggestive of infection and a doctor should be consulted.

Eye strain, due to refractive errors, and nasal congestion or sinusitis may cause headaches. When a child is experiencing frequent bad headaches, parents often worry about the possibility of a brain tumour or other neurological problems. Tumours are rare in childhood and seldom present with a headache as the main symptom.

Children who have sustained a head injury may have intermittent headaches for some months afterwards, even though there is no residual damage from the original injury. Other causes of headache in childhood are uncommon.

Migraine and stress headaches

In some people the blood vessels of the scalp and the brain constrict and dilate more readily than in other people, and having this increased reactivity of the vessels of the head makes them liable to develop migraine headaches. The tendency to migraine often runs in families. An episode of spasm of these blood vessels may be provoked by intense concentration or by stress, by eating certain foods to which they are sensitive, and often by unknown factors. The result is a bad headache,

Migraine

It is not known why particular individuals are susceptible to migraine headaches, but in those who are, bright lights, noise, or stress may provoke an attack. It is also thought that certain foods, notably coffee, cheese and chocolate may precipitate an attack. It may be advisable to avoid these foods if there seems to be a connection with attacks.

The symptoms of migraine vary from child to child, but often the first features of an attack are visual disturbance such as seeing zigzags or flashing lights. This may be followed by nausea as well as headache.

If you think that your child has a migraine attack coming on, or he gets the first symptoms, splashing the face with cold water (below), giving any prescribed medications and letting him lie down in a darkened room may all help to alleviate the attack.

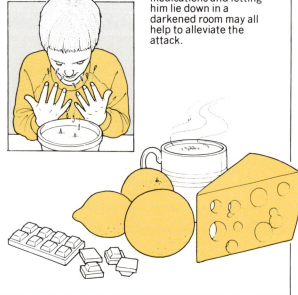

Headaches caused by worry or fatigue, the most common kind, may arise from tension of the muscles of the neck and scalp. With migraine, the arteries leading to the brain constrict and dilate, causing a disturbance in the blood flow to the brain. This narrowing of the arteries is the result of a spasm of the muscle in the wall of the artery, as shown in the diagram on the right.

The factors which lead to arterial spasm in migraine sufferers differ between individuals but may include nervous tension and food allergies.

Normal artery (diagramatic)

Media This is the muscular layer of the artery, with smooth muscle cells arranged in a circular way around the artery

Adventitia This is the outer layer of the artery and consists of fibrous tissue

Intima This is the layer which lines the artery, consisting of endothelial cells.

Artery in spasm with muscular contraction narrowing the vessel.

often accompanied by visual disturbance such as seeing flashing lights, and by nausea and/or vomiting.

Young children do not often get migraine headaches, but some children who have recurrent abdominal pain in mid-childhood go on to develop migraine instead in late childhood or adolescence.

Both concentration and anxiety give rise to excessive and sometimes prolonged contraction of the muscles of the neck and scalp, and this may lead on to so-called stress headaches. The cause may be readily apparent, as in the child whose headache comes on after studying hard at some difficult homework, or it may be less obvious.

The distinction between stress headaches and migraine is not always clear, and in practice is often not important. When a child complains of a headache it may be enough to have a short break with a drink or biscuit to allow it to pass off. If the headache persists, paracetamol or soluble aspirin may bring relief, or lying down in a quiet room may help.

If a child is getting frequent severe headaches, it suggests there is underlying stress or anxiety which may be acting as a precipitant. Common reasons for stress at school include teasing or bullying, a teacher who is feared or disliked, or being unable to understand or keep up with schoolwork. At home, children often come under stress when there is marital discord, when somebody in the family is ill, or if a move of house is being contemplated. Financial and other worries within the household are also sensed by children, and may give rise to stress symptoms. When headaches are frequent and causing serious interference in a child's lifestyle, enquiries should be made at school into any possible problems, and the doctor should be consulted.

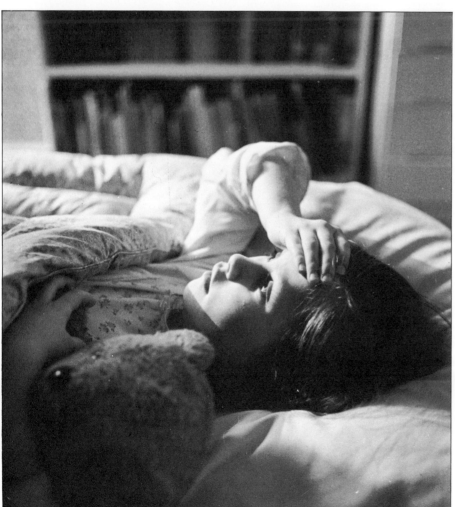

Mild headaches are not uncommon in childhood and they are usually alleviated by rest, and treatment with analgesics such as aspirin or paracetamol. They can be caused by physical factors, such as eye strain, noise, lack of sleep, over exertion or concentration, or they may arise as a result of worry or tension.

Relaxation and rest is the best remedy, so if your child is suffering from a headache, give him a mild analgesic and put him to bed in a darkened room.

If your child has frequent headaches or migraine attacks, you should ask your doctor's advice about treatment.

Behavioural problems

CHILDREN HAVE TO LEARN how they are expected to behave from those around them, particularly from their parents. It takes time for them to learn what is, and what is not, acceptable behaviour, and some children take longer than others. Disturbances of behaviour may occur because of delayed learning, as a reaction to anxieties and adverse situations or during a period of adaptation to new circumstances.

THE PRE-SCHOOL CHILD
Sleeping problems

Problems with a child waking during the night, or having difficulty in getting to sleep in the evening are very common. Some infants and young children do not establish a routine of sleeping through the night until the age of three or four. They wake once, or even several times a night, and although often they will settle when turned over, or on hearing a reassuring voice or being given a drink, sometimes they will be wakeful and demand prolonged adult attention.

This does not indicate that anything is wrong with the child. It is a variant of normal behaviour, but if the pattern is repeated night after night, the parents become sleep deprived, and may be tired, irritable and have less tolerance than usual during the day. Under these circumstances, the emotional stability of the family becomes threatened.

Sedatives are often prescribed in this situation, but seldom help a lot. Most mild sedatives which are suitable for children only last for a few hours so, if given at bedtime, have worn off by the middle of the night. Furthermore, regular sedative medication of children is generally undesirable. Instead the family organization may have to change, so that the parents can spend longer in bed to catch up on sleep, or can arrange to have an occasional 'night off' with the child staying at a grandparent's or friend's. For some couples, having the baby in their own bed is a reasonable compromise. Fortunately as the child matures the sleep pattern is likely to change so that the repeated waking ceases.

The child who has difficulty in getting off to sleep is often emotionally wound up at bedtime. This can be because the day has been full, exciting and challenging, or can be because of insecurity or emotional upset. In either case, a period of calm and ordered routine for a couple of hours before bedtime, with plenty of affection and comfort, is likely to be helpful. Unfortunately the parents' anxiety, aroused by the knowledge that getting off to sleep can be difficult, acts against a period of calm and stability at bedtime, so that a vicious circle is set up.

Overactive and attention-seeking behaviour

Young children enjoy activities with adults, whether playing games, helping with housework, or shopping.

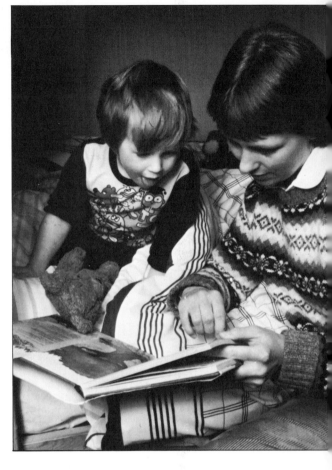

This interaction is very important for learning and development. When toddler-aged children are left to their own devices, they only perform the task for a short period before changing to something else, or seeking adult attention. They seem to be always on the go, so looking after small children can be very demanding.

This short attention span is normal in toddlers, but as they grow older concentration normally improves, and the pre-school child will often be busy with toys or tasks for long periods without needing the attention or intervention of anyone else. A child with a short attention span will seldom be still for any length of time, so will appear overactive. There is some discrepancy in attention span and activity among normal children, but other factors may also affect concentration. Children with mental handicap may appear overactive as their behaviour is more in keeping with their developmental age than their normal age. Children who are insecure or otherwise emotionally disturbed are likely to have only limited concentration, in the same way that anxious adults can seldom sit still for long. If a child seeks adult attention which is not immediately forthcoming, the

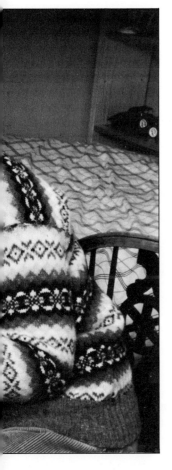

Some children dislike going to bed, others have difficulty in getting off to sleep, while others wake during the night. Generally these problems do not indicate that there is anything wrong with the child, but they can cause upset for the parents. A child who will not sleep at night prevents parents from getting an adequate amount of sleep too, and no one can function well if they are continually tired. There is no easy way of coping with a child who will not sleep at night, but sometimes establishing a routine at bedtime can ease the problem. The child can be read a story or sung a song in bed at night and this might help to calm him and make him sleepy. However some children do not seem to respond to this kind of routine. In these cases, anything which is found to help is acceptable. This may include being flexible about the time a child goes to bed, having a cot in the parents' room, or even sleeping in the parents' bed.

and severe mental handicap are normally identified in early childhood, there is no clear border between dull children and those with mild mental handicap. The inability to learn adequately in a normal school should be the major criterion in deciding whether a dull child needs special education, and this may not become apparent until the school acknowledges that there is a learning problem.

Children of normal and above average intelligence may have learning difficulties in school. These may be because unsuspected physical handicaps, visual impairment due to refractive errors, or partial hearing loss have passed unnoticed in the home. Severe colour blindness may lead to difficulty if concepts are taught utilizing colour as one of the discriminating factors. Tests of vision and hearing may be indicated in a child with unexpected learning difficulties.

Children who are anxious or emotionally insecure may have difficulty in learning. Such anxiety can arise within the home, if there is marital discord or separation, unemployment, financial difficulty, or other stresses. Even though parents may try to minimize the effect of such events on their children, inevitably they will be aware of tensions within the family and be affected by them.

The anxiety may arise at school. Some teachers appear frightening to a child, or there may be teasing or bullying from other children. School lavatories often cause anxiety for children. Furthermore, if a child is having difficulty in learning this, in itself, can cause distress for the child.

child may become more insistent in his or her demands. When parental attention is distracted the child may become exasperated and awkward. He may be naughty to provoke a reaction when other demands have failed. To a child in this state, being told off may be preferable to being apparently ignored.

Some children who are otherwise normal in their behaviour may appear to be more active than their peers, and have less good concentration. This can cause problems in a nursery or a school setting, as well as in the family. The name hyperactivity syndrome has been applied to such behaviour. Attempts have been made to explain the hyperactivity syndrome both on the basis of minimal brain damage, and on possible toxic effects of various foods and food additives. There is little convincing evidence yet that it represents more than one extreme of the wide range of normal child behaviour.

THE SCHOOL CHILD
Learning difficulties
Children may have difficulty in learning because their intelligence is below the average. Although moderate

Dyslexia
In addition to intellectual impairment, physical handicap and emotional disorders, some children have difficulty in learning to read and write because of a specific learning disorder sometimes known as dyslexia. Dyslexia may be of varying severity, and is often familial. It is more common in boys than in girls, and when present to a mild degree may be indistinguishable from other causes of poor learning. In a more severe form, there appears to be a major problem in reading, in forming letters and words and in grasping the basic concepts of written language, while verbal use of intelligence can be above average, and skills with numbers may be unimpaired. With persistence, remedial help, and increasing motivation, children with specific reading difficulty will usually learn to read and write, but may continue to have problems with spelling and written fluency.

School Phobia and truancy
School phobia is a state of anxiety in a child induced either by going to school, or because of a fear of leaving home. It can come on at any age, and is usually

Stress in Childhood

The Pre-school child		The school child	
Causes	Manifestations	Causes	Manifestations
Family anxieties	Poor feeding	Family anxieties	Poor learning
Marital disharmony	Continual crying	Marital disharmony	Sleep disturbance
Emotional deprivation	Clinging behaviour	Emotional deprivation	Difficult behaviour
Social stress • Parental unemployment • Poor housing • Financial stringency	Attention-seeking behaviour Sleep disturbance Hyperactivity	Social stress	Tantrums
		Mental illness in the family	Tearfulness
		Moving house	Abdominal pain
Mental illness in the family		Sibling rivalry	Headaches
Moving house		Disablity or handicap	School phobia
Sibling rivalry		Insecurity	Truancy
Disablity or handicap		Bullying and teasing	Stealing
		Anxieties about self and achievements	Solvent abuse
		Apprehensions over pubertal development, sex, attractiveness, gender role, career, examinations	Anorexia Delinquency

manifested in the development of symptoms such as severe headaches, abdominal pain, nausea or feeling faint. This will lead to the child being kept at home or being sent home from school.

The symptoms are usually thought to indicate an underlying illness, but there may be a periodicity about them which is suggestive. Symptoms may be worse first thing in the morning, mainly on weekdays, and better during school holidays. However, in many children the symptoms can occur at any time because the underlying anxiety is present much of the time.

School phobia is seldom due to one single underlying factor, more to an accumulation of factors which induce the anxiety state. The factors at school which may contribute are dislike or fear of a teacher, an inability to do some, or all, of the school work, fear of ridicule, poor relationships with other children, or teasing and bullying. Teasing by other children can be very cruel and is often based on some individual peculiarity such as obesity, wearing glasses, or coming from a different background, which itself becomes a source of anxiety for the child. Apparent school phobia may in fact be due to a fear of leaving home, either because home is percieved as a safe place or because tensions within the home and family may have induced an insecurity, making the child feel he must be there to know what is happening, or to prevent family breakdown.

Once school phobia is established and the child has missed some schooling, he or she is likely to get behind with school work. This may induce further anxiety. Furthermore, the longer the child is away, the less easy the social integration with the other children will be. As a consequence, the child becomes more individual, and separate from the group.

The child's distress is likely to lead the parent to want to keep him away from school, or alternatively, the school may send the child home because of the repeated headaches and other symptoms. Although this seems reasonable in the short term, it perpetuates the problem. Unless these anxieties are faced and overcome, they are likely to persist and get worse.

Minor incidence of school phobia is common, and can be handled by the sympathetic parent calmly and firmly, perhaps with some cooperation from the school. More severe school phobia may require the help of a child psychiatrist to help in its resolution.

Truancy, taking time off from school without consent, is common on an occasional basis in adolescence. If it becomes regular or persistent, it may indicate social isolation and insecurity. Furthermore, children who play truant may drift into other misdemeanors which can bring them into conflict with society and the law. The truant child needs help with any underlying problems and firmness in handling the truancy.

Anorexia nervosa

MOST TEENAGE GIRLS ARE interested in their weight and appearance, and 'going on a diet' is accepted as normal adolescent behaviour. Anorexia nervosa is a psychological disturbance, almost exclusively confined to females, in which a girl feels she is too fat and then develops a compulsion to lose weight.

Some affected people are plump or fat at the onset of the disease, but many are not. One of the characteristics of anorexia nervosa is the persistent feeling of being too fat, even if it is recognized at the same time by the patient that she is thinner than other girls of her age.

With the development of this weight phobia, the food intake is progressively restricted, with particular avoidance of starchy and sugary foods. Weight is gradually lost, and in severe cases the affected person can become seriously wasted. When weight loss is extreme, menstruation ceases, there may be increased growth of hair on the body, and the hands and feet are usually cold.

Anorexia nervosa most commonly starts between the ages of 15 and 16 years, but may start as early as 11 years. Minor symptoms of the condition are very common. The girl constantly keeps an eye on her diet even though she appears to her family and friends to be thin.

The underlying personality difficulties which lead to the development of anorexia nervosa are complex, different in each patient, and may not be easy to determine. In some patients a reluctance to accept becoming a woman with all that it implies — changing body shape,

menstruation, relationships with the opposite sex, marriage and pregnancy — may be a factor. With severe anorexia, breasts waste away and periods stop; puberty in fact will seem to be arrested or may even regress.

Stresses within the family may be a contributory factor. Often the family has high expectations for the girl's future, and worry about exams or a career may be present. Whatever the originating problems, they tend to become pushed into the background as the girl becomes obsessed with food, body weight, and dieting. In patients with severe anorexia nervosa, induced vomiting and frequent use of laxatives are common. These, together with the emaciation that can result from the self-induced starvation, can become life threatening.

If anorexia is suspected the doctor should be consulted. It may be necessary to do some tests to exclude other diseases as a cause for the wasting, but often the diagnosis can be made on history and examination alone. In mild cases it may be enough to keep a regular eye on the weight to make sure it does not get too low, as there is a tendency to spontaneous improvement as the girl gets older. In more severe cases, there is a dual approach to treatment; refeeding until a target weight is attained, together with an attempt to identify and resolve inner personality conflicts and difficulties which have led to the development of the condition. A psychiatrist will need to supervize treatment and, if weight loss has been severe, hospitalization may be necessary. In severe cases treatment and support may need to be prolonged.

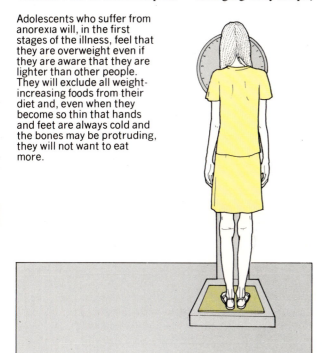

Adolescents who suffer from anorexia will, in the first stages of the illness, feel that they are overweight even if they are aware that they are lighter than other people. They will exclude all weight-increasing foods from their diet and, even when they become so thin that hands and feet are always cold and the bones may be protruding, they will not want to eat more.

Treatment of Anorexia Nervosa

The treatment of anorexia nervosa includes increasing the food intake until an adequate weight is achieved, together with pyschiatric treatment to help to resolve underlying emotional problems.

In severe cases admission to hospital is necessary, and the patient may have to be restricted in her activities until she is eating more. Great skill may be required by the nurses to achieve an adequate food intake, and supervision is needed to avoid self-induced vomiting after meals.

Drugs are sometimes given to relax inner tensions and anxieties, but resolving the inner personality conflicts is necessary for complete cure. Particulary common are anxieties over

growing up, including achieving independence from parents, personal relationships, and attaining physical maturity.

Although many patients improve rapidly, in severe cases prolonged treatment will be needed.

The eyes

NORMAL VISION IMPLIES the ability to see clearly, to be able to distinguish fine detail, and to perceive small objects. In addition to this high acuity, normal vision also includes the ability to focus close-up, to be able to see both in very bright light and in dull conditions, to be able to appreciate different colours, and to use both eyes together to appreciate distance.

To fulfil these various functions, the structure and function of the eyes is necessarily complex. Each eye is approximately spherical and is held in place inside a protective bony socket by fine muscles. These muscles are controlled by nerves which ensure that the eyes move in unison. The outside of the eyeball consists of tough white fibrous tissue called the sclera. At the front there is

a circular clear area, the cornea, which lets the light into the eye. The front of the eye is covered with a protective layer of delicate membrane called the conjunctiva which also lines the inside of the eyelids. Immediately behind the cornea is the iris which constricts and dilates to control the amount of light entering the eye, and behind the iris is the lens.

The lens focuses the light onto the back of the eye, forming clear images of what is being looked at. Muscles inside the eye can alter the lens to enable it to focus on near objects. The back of the eye is lined with the retina, which is a light sensitive layer. Some of the cells of the retina, the cones, are concerned with colour vision and high acuity, while others, the rods, are more responsive

The eye is set in a protective bony socket lined with fatty tissue and is held in place by three pairs of strong muscles. The thick outer layer of the eye, the sclera surrounds the eyeball except for the transparent window at the front called the cornea. The conjunctiva covers the outer surface of the cornea and the inner surface of the lids. Behind the cornea is the iris and behind the iris is the lens.

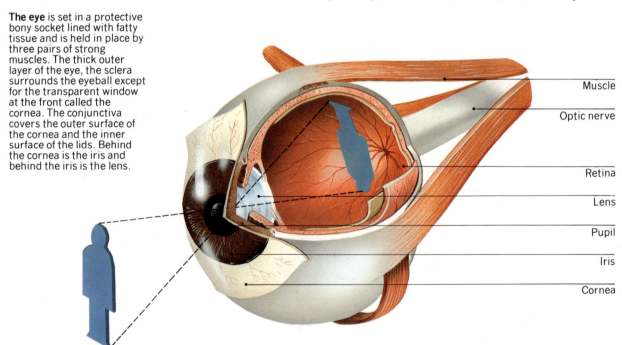

Muscle

Optic nerve

Retina

Lens

Pupil

Iris

Cornea

The image above Light reflected from an object enters the eye through the transparent cornea. The lens then focuses the light onto the back of the eye, forming a clear image of what is being looked at. The lens also turns the image upside down (see above). On the retina, which lines the back of the eye, are millions of cells called rods and cones; these cells convert the rays of light into electrical impulses and send them via the optic nerve to the brain.

Visual pathways to the brain

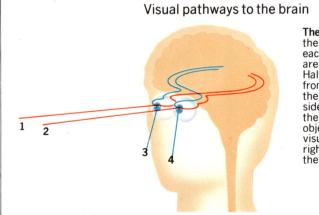

1
2
3
4

The eye Two visual centres in the brain, one at the back of each cerebral hemisphere, are responsible for sight. Half the optic nerve fibres from each eye cross over to the visual centre on the other side of the brain. Therefore the left visual centre 'sees' objects in the right half of the visual field (1, 2) and the right centre 'sees' objects in the left half (3, 4).

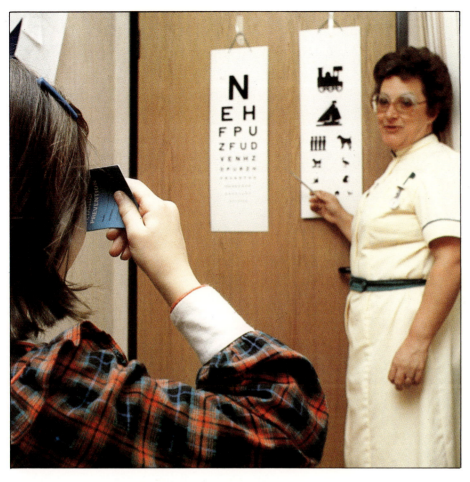

Every few years a child should have an eye test. The visual acuity of pre-school children can be tested by asking them to match letters, even if they do not know the alphabet. Older children are asked to identify letters from a wall chart or flash card.

in dim light. These cells send impulses via the optic nerve to the brain. The brain then reinterprets these impulses into the visual images perceived by the individual.

Eye tests for children

When the doctor examines the eye he looks in turn at the eye movements, the conjunctiva, the cornea, the iris, the lens, and the retina. Eye movements are tested by making the child look in different directions. The conjunctiva is readily visible. If it appears red and inflamed, the doctor will diagnose conjunctivitis. By shining a light into the eye, the doctor can see if the iris is working by watching the pupil constrict. The cornea and lens are normally transparent, and the doctor looks through them with an opthalmoscope. Any opacity will call for further investigation. With the opthalmoscope the doctor can see the retina and its blood vessels, and the beginning of the optic nerve. Sometimes it is necessary to put drops into the eye to dilate the pupil to assist the examination.

Vision testing in small children may be difficult. At a few weeks old a child should be able to follow with his eyes a face or moving toy nearby. Watching an infant playing with a toy or picking up objects may help in assessing visual ability. When the child is a toddler, visual acuity can be tested reasonably accurately using different sized white balls at different distances. Older children can identify or match letters from a wall chart or flash card.

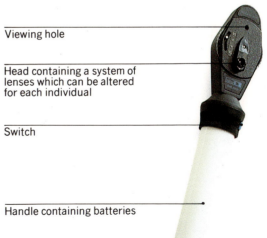

Viewing hole

Head containing a system of lenses which can be altered for each individual

Switch

Handle containing batteries

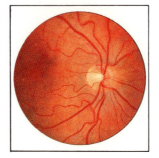

With the ophthalmoscope (see above) the doctor can see the retina and its blood vessels, and the beginning of the optic nerve (left).

Refractive errors and visual disturbances

Short sightedness In short sightedness, or myopia, the lens of the eye focuses in front of the retina. The image of the retina is blurred for all objects except those close to it. A concave lens corrects the refractive error giving a normal range of vision.

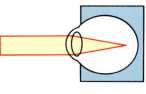

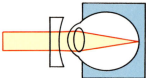

Long sightedness In long sightedness, or hypermetropia, the lens of the eye tends to focus behind the retina and only distant objects can be seen clearly. A corrective convex lens restores a normal range of vision.

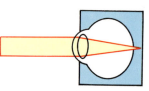

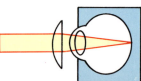

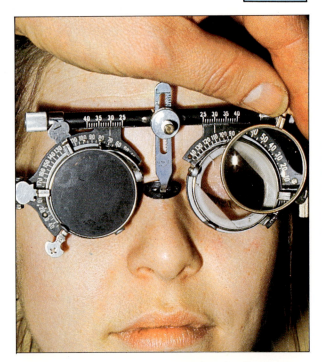

The optician puts in a combination of different lenses until he finds which one is best for the child. The combination resulting in the sharpest image is called the refractive error.

Once the refractive error is found the child can be fitted with suitable lenses. The success of this kind of test depends upon reliable responses from the child.

IN A PERSON WITH normal vision, the resting eye is in focus for distant objects. The eye will adjust to focus on near objects by the contraction of ciliary muscles which alter the shape of the lens. If the resting eye is focused on near objects the individual is said to be short-sighted or myopic, and will be unable to see distant objects clearly. A person who cannot focus on near objects, is said to be long-sighted, or hypermetropic.

At birth most children are far-sighted, that is they cannot focus clearly on near objects. This is because the eye is small and the lens focuses behind the retina. This usually corrects during the first year but some children remain hypermetropic.

Children with refractive errors are not aware of their disability. They may have a squint, or show lack of interest in books or in television, or may tire easily when they are concentrating on close work. Any child who is suspected of having a refractive problem should be properly assessed.

Hypermetropia (far-sightedness)

The hypermetropic eye is shorter than normal and therefore hypermetropia tends to be a problem in early childhood. The child may be able to see close work by adjusting, but the continued use of the ciliary muscles leads to fatigue and possibly headache. Hypermetropia can be corrected by a convex lens, which helps the eye to focus on the retina at close distances without strain. If only one eye is hypermetropic this may interfere with binocular vision, and a squint may result.

Myopia (short-sightedness)

In myopia the eyeball is longer than normal, and the lens focuses in front of the retina. Myopia is usually manifest in mid-childhood, with the child being unable to read the blackboard, or see distant objects. Myopia is often familial. Spectacles with concave lenses will correct the refractive error. The myopia can be progressive for a few years, so the eyes need regular testing in case the corrective lenses need altering.

Astigmatism

In astigmatism there is an irregularity either in the lens or in the shape of the eyeball, so that an irregular image is produced. Slight astigmatism is common, and seldom needs correction, but a more severe condition will require glasses to be worn some, or all, of the time. Astigmatism may be associated with myopia or hypermetropia.

Squints

One of the skills that babies have to learn in the early months of life is the ability to use both eyes together for looking at an object — a necessary skill for judging distances and preventing double vision. A squint (or strabismus) is when the eyes do not move together, and this is common in childhood. Transient squints noted in babies are usually unimportant, being due to immaturity in coordination. Persistent squints, and those present after about three months, are likely to be significant, and require an expert opinion on whether or not treatment is necessary.

In most childhood squints the defect is in the eyes moving together. There may be full movement of each eye separately, but whichever direction the child looks in a squint is noticeable. Usually the eyes are turned in towards each other. This is known as a concomitant squint, and may be due to a minor defect in development in which the muscles that move the eye are slightly in the wrong position. Such defects are readily correctable by surgery, and if done early, results are very good, although for marked squints more than one operation is needed. Concomitant squints also occur because of defective vision in one or both eyes. If the visual defect can be corrected with spectacles the squint may right itself.

Squints may be due to defective vision, but a concomitant squint can also cause a visual defect in one eye. If the eyes do not move in unison they see slightly different things, and this can result in double vision. In young children the brain 'switches off' the image from one eye. This eliminates the double vision, but can eventually lead to loss of function of one eye, so-called amblyopia or 'lazy eye'.

This 'lazy eye' must be made to work again before any operation to correct the squint is performed. This is done by covering the 'good' eye with a patch for some months until full vision returns to the 'lazy eye'. Beyond the age of seven years it is rare for sight to recover in amblyopic eyes, emphasizing the need for early diagnosis and treatment of squints.

When there is paralysis of one or more of the muscles which move the eye, a different sort of squint occurs. The squint is variable, and is not noticeable when the child is looking in one direction, but marked when looking in another. Such paralytic squints are uncommon in children. When they occur they may be due to a developmental anomaly or to a disease of the eye. An opthalmic opinion is needed to decide on the cause and necessary treatment.

Children who at first glance are thought to have a squint, are occasionally seen, on closer examination, to have eyes that are straight and move together. The appearance of a squint in these children is due to asymmetry of the bridge of the nose, or of the skinfolds at the inner angle of the eyes. No treatment is necessary and the apparent squint becomes less pronounced as the child grows. In almost all children with squints, treatment is

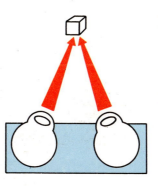

Normal In looking at distant objects the axis of each eye is normally parallel. On looking at close objects the movements of the two eyes are coordinated so that both look at the same thing. This gives a three dimensional appreciation of the object and assessment of its distance away.

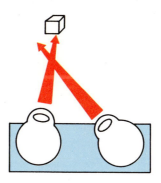

Convergent squint With a convergent squint, the axis of each eye is not coordinated so that both eyes are directed to the object, but the axes cross in front of the object giving the eyes a cross-eyed appearance.

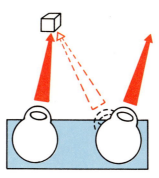

Divergent squint With a divergent squint the eyes do not move together. One eye is turned outwards so that the axes of the eyes diverge.

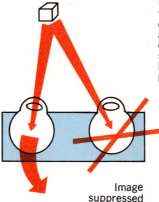

Lazy eye In young children with squints the image from one eye is often suppressed, and this is known as a lazy eye, or ambylopia. If the squint is not corrected the lazy eye may become permanently non-functional.

Image suppressed

How the eye moves The eyeball moves from side to side and up and down, because of the pull of attached muscles. There are six muscles attached to the globe of each eye, and to the surrounding orbit. The coordinated contraction of these muscles (far right) moves the eye to look up and down (3) or sideways (2), or to oblique positions in between (1). Normally these movements are coordinated so that the two eyes move together. With a squint the coordination between the movements of the eyes is defective, as in the boy on the right. It may be possible to correct this by an operation.

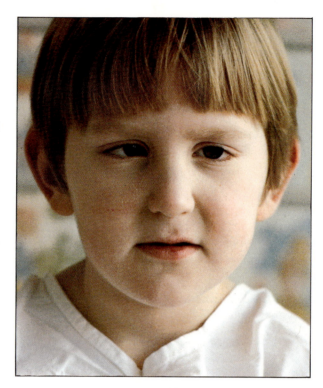

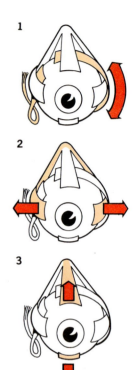

possible to correct the defect. It is important that an expert opinion is obtained early so that optimal treatment can be planned.

Visual disturbances

A child's vision may be impaired in various ways. The eyes may not focus properly at all distances unless appropriate spectacles are worn. This is known as refractive error. The eyes may not coordinate together all the time to give binocular vision (using both eyes) because of a squint, or the appreciation of colour may be impaired due to *colour blindness*.

The most serious visual handicaps are due to loss of acuity leading to partial sightedness or blindness. Such problems are fortunately uncommon, but may be due to a variety of conditions, and different parts of the visual pathway can be affected. Scarring of the cornea, opacity of the lens (cataract), retinal disease, pressure or damage to the optic nerve, or damage to the occipital part of the brain that interprets visual impulses coming from the eyes, can all lead to varying degreees of visual handicap.

Cataracts and damage to the cornea can usually be treated, but visual handicap as a result of damage to the retina or occipital part of the brain is usually permanent. An expert ophthalmological opinion is required for any child thought to be visually handicapped. Children with serious visual handicaps need special learning and

Eye illnesses

Eye infections are not unusual in childhood and rarely cause serious problems. Inflammation of the eyelids and of the conjunctiva, the transparent lining of the lid, are the most common and can usually be treated at home.

Styes A stye is a localized infection in the hair follicle of the eyelash. It resembles a small boil on the eyelid and is uncomfortable rather than painful.

The stye can be treated at home with ointment prescribed by the doctor or by applying heat to the inflamed area. This can be done by holding a flannel, soaked in hot salty water, to the stye for a few minutes. This increases the blood supply to the infected part and enables it to clear more rapidly.

Most children have the occasional stye, but if your child gets them repeatedly you should consult your doctor.

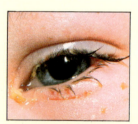

The picture above shows a child with cellulitis of the lids. This is inflammation of the cellular tissue, commonly caused by infection. It can be treated effectively with drugs

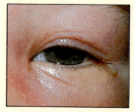

Conjunctivitis (above) is inflammation of the conjunctiva, due to infection with bacteria or viruses. It responds to treatment with antibiotics.

developmental stimulation from an early age to learn communicative skills, and to minimize the consequences of their handicap.

Colour blindness

Although children are often unable to name colours until about the age of three, their appreciation of colour begins long before this. Bright colours attract children, and many can match bricks for colour long before they can name them individually.

A total inability to appreciate differences in colour is excessively rare, but some degree of difficulty in distinguishing between colours, so-called colour blindness, is very common. Colour blindness is a genetic disorder which is manifested mainly in males. About eight per cent of boys have some degree of colour blindness, whereas it only affects about one girl in every 500.

Colour blindness can be of varying severity. In essence it consists of a difficulty in distinguishing shades of colour which most people recognize as being different. Most colour-blind individuals have no difficulty in distinguishing between red, orange, yellow, green and blue, but they may have great difficulty in discriminating between, for instance, lime green, emerald green and turquoise, or between varying shades of red. If the colour blindness is mild, it may pass completely unnoticed even into adult life, and may cause either no practical difficulties, or nothing worse than choosing clothes which do not precisely match.

For those few occupations in which even mild degrees of colour blindness may be a disadvantage (such as pilots or train drivers) tests of colour vision are part of the medical examination.

Severe colour blindness may be apparent during childhood, but as with other handicaps such as visual loss or hearing defect, the child himself does not realize there is a disability. This puts the onus for recognition of the disability onto those who care for children. Many toys and teaching aids, such as beads, bricks and counting rods, rely on colour to emphasize the different types. A child with impaired colour perception who is taught with colour-coded aids may seem to be having more than average difficulty in learning. Frequently this will manifest itself in lack of attentiveness, fidgeting or naughtiness. It is easy to get cross with the child, or seek an emotional cause for the learning difficulty and bad behaviour, when the real explanation may be colour blindness.

If colour blindness is suspected, tests for defective colour vision can be done, either by using specially designed coloured number charts, or else by matching coloured wools with a test card.

Provided colour blindness is recognized in childhood, alternative teaching methods can be used.

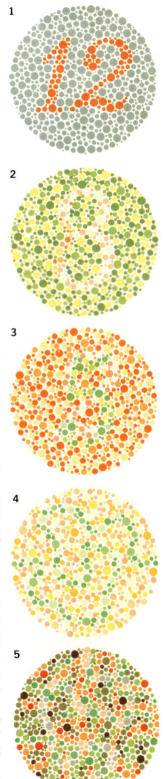

Colour defective vision
People with colour defective vision fall into two main groups. Protanopes, those in the most common group, find it difficult to distinguish between red, orange, yellow and green. Eye specialists believe that the retina of a protanope (the layer of light-sensitive cells at the back of the eye) has too few of the cone cells responsible for absorbing red light. Protanopes, therefore, have to distinguish the whole spectrum of colours using only 'green-sensitive' and 'blue-sensitive' cone cells.

Deuteranopes, those in the second group, lack cones responsible for absorbing green light. Like protanopes, they tend to confuse red, orange, yellow and green, but they see green and yellow as shades of red and brown.

To test for colour defective vision, a colour confusion test is carried out under carefully controlled lighting conditions. The examples here should not be used for self-diagnosis.

Children with normal vision and those with all types of defective vision see, in **example 1**, the number 12.

In **example 2** children with normal vision see the number 8 — those with a red-green defect will see the number 3. Those with total colour defective vision cannot see a numeral at all.

In **example 3** children with normal vision see the number 5. Those with a red-green defect see the number 2 and those with total defect cannot see a numeral.

For the next test the child will be asked to connect the winding line of green dots in **example 4**. Any child with total defect cannot see a line at all.

Whether the child has normal colour vision or defective colour vision, he will not be able to see a numeral in **example 5**. This is because there is no numeral — it is a trick test.

The skin and birthmarks

A CHILD'S SKIN IS soft and delicate, but nevertheless forms a tough flexible covering for the body. The skin helps to protect the body from infection, controls heat loss, and will develop protective pigmentation if exposed to the sun. The skin is also a major sense organ, being able to appreciate temperature, touch, pressure and pain.

Under the microscope the skin can be seen to consist of two main layers; the outer epidermis and the dermis below. The epidermis is the waterproof layer and consists of cells with thick walls of a tough protein called keratin. This layer also contains the pigment cells which produce pigment in response to ultra violent irradiation, such as sunlight. The dermis contains blood vessels and nerves, as well as fibrous tissue to give both strength and flexibility. In addition, sweat glands, hair roots and follicles are in the dermal layer.

When injured, skin usually heals rapidly, so that most cuts and abrasions will be better within a week or so. If only the epidermis is involved no scarring takes place, but when the dermis is injured a scar may result. With cuts, healing is quicker and the scarring is less if the wound edges are held together. Large wounds or gaping incisions heal better if they are stitched.

Birthmarks

Unusual marks on the skin of newborn babies are known as naevi, or birthmarks. They consist either of an area of abnormal pigmentation, or of a localized abnormality of the blood vessels in the skin. They vary widely in size and position; some are unsightly, but many are insignificant, or even give an individuality which is a source of pride. The different sorts of birthmarks have different names, and knowing the type of mark will often enable the doctor to tell what will happen to it.

Stork Marks

Many newborn babies have a distinctive triangular blotchy red mark arising between the eyebrows and spreading out over the forehead. There is almost always an accompanying red patch at the back of the neck. The name derives from the fanciful notion that they are caused by the stork delivering the baby's head in its beak. Although stork marks may be prominent in infancy, they gradually fade and do not persist into childhood.

Strawberry Marks

Although not usually present at birth, as they appear in the first month of life, strawberry marks are generally classed as birthmarks. They can occur anywhere on the skin, and consist of localized dilatation of blood vessels giving rise to a bright red, raised bumpy lesion. The name strawberry mark is more descriptive of their appearance than the alternative, cavernous haemangioma. Strawberry marks may go on enlarging until the

The skin is strong, soft and flexible and protects the body. It consists of two main layers, the epidermis on the outside and the dermis underneath.

The outer layer of the epidermis is made up of hardened cells which gradually flake off, but are replaced by new cells growing from the lower layers of the epidermis. In these lower epidermal layers the skin pigment is produced which determines the colour of the skin.

The dermis contains the sweat glands and the hair follicles, and their associated sebaceous glands which produce the natural greases which keep the skin supple and waterproof and help to protect against infection.

Nerve ending

Vein

Dermis

Artery

Epidermis

Sebaceous gland

Hair

Muscle attached to hair follicle

Sweat gland

Hair follicle

Fat

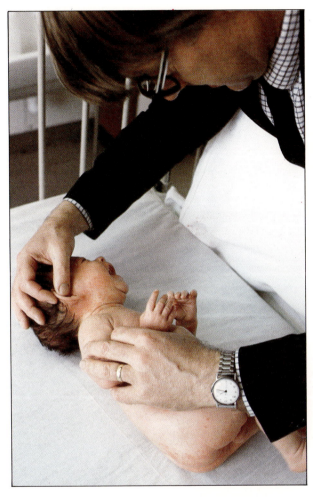

A dermatologist is a doctor who specialises in the diagnosis and treatment of disorders of the skin. The doctor in the illustration is examining a baby with seborrhoeic eczema. Birthmarks, sometimes called naevi, are of many different forms. Those shown here (below) are the most common, but there are other types.

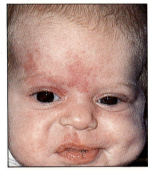

Stork Mark

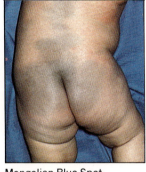

Strawberry Mark

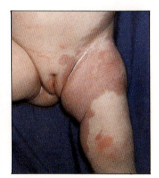

Mongolian Blue Spot

Port Wine Stain

child is about six months old, and may become quite extensive. They may be unsightly if they involve the face, they can bleed if they get knocked, and occasionally they become infected. Beyond the age of about six to nine months, there is no further enlargement, but instead a gradual reduction in size occurs until they disappear altogether. They have always gone by about the age of five years, leaving virtually no trace.

There is no treatment effective in speeding their departure which does not carry some risk of permanent scarring, so these marks are best left alone.

Café-au-lait spots
One of the commonest forms of naevi are smooth light brown patches of skin occurring anywhere on the body. They are seldom unsightly and persist throughout life.

Mongolian Blue spots
Babies of Asian, African, or West Indian origin, may have a bluish discoloration of the lower back, sometimes spreading as far up as the shoulders. This gradually becomes less obvious as the child grows up. These marks were once thought only to occur in Chinese babies, hence the name Mongolian blue spots.

Port Wine Stains
Much less common than strawberry marks are the so-called port wine stains, which are irregularly shaped deep red patches on the skin. They consist of dilated capillaries in the skin filled with blood. They persist throughout life, are usually small, but can be extensive, and attempted removal leads to scarring. There are, however, preliminary reports suggesting that laser treatment can help.

Other birthmarks
Other forms of birthmarks are occasionally seen. For any birthmark which is unsightly or causing anxiety, the opinion of a dermatologist should be sought, and advice obtained on the most appropriate form of treatment.

Common skin disorders in infancy

ECZEMA IS AN INFLAMED red rash common in babies and children. There are two different forms of eczema, seborrhoeic eczema and atopic eczema, which, although similar in appearance, are different in character and prognosis, so will be described separately.

Seborrhoeic Eczema

This may begin in the newborn period, within a few days of birth. Red inflamed areas appear on the skin creases of the groin and buttocks, behind the ears, and on the scalp and neck and in the armpits. There is often an associated greasy scaley area on the scalp, the so-called 'cradle cap'. The rash does not seem to irritate or distress the baby, but from time to time it may become more extensive or become infected. Seborrhoeic eczema responds readily to treatment with a mild steroid cream, and does not recur after infancy.

Atopic Eczema

This first appears between the ages of about two months and two years. There may be a history of eczema, asthma or hay fever in a close relative, as these three are the principle manifestations of the ATOPIC SYNDROME, which is often familial.

A red, itchy rash develops in patches, particularly on the limbs and cheeks, but other areas may be involved. At first the rash may show vesicles or small blisters, which weep clear fluid if they are scratched, and later the skin becomes thickened and scaly. As the child gets older, the rash becomes less extensive. In some children it clears completely after infancy, but in others it persists throughout childhood, and is mainly confined to the flexures of wrist, elbows, knees, and ankles.

In some patients, eczema is aggravated by allergies to food products. In severe eczema it may be worth trying a diet which avoids milk, eggs and dairy products. This should only be done under medical guidance, and to make sure that the diet is not nutritionally deficient.

Continuous skin care in eczema helps to prevent aggravation of the rash. Soap which tends to dry the skin is best avoided, and an emulsifying ointment should be used instead. Emulsifying ointments soften the skin and prevent it flaking. The whole skin can be treated by putting some ointment in the bathwater.

When patches of eczema do develop, prompt treatment with a mild steroid cream will usually relieve itching and settle the rash. Scratching aggravates the rash, and should be avoided. Fingernails should be cut short, and if the child scratches whilst asleep, mittens should be worn in bed. Nocturnal itching may be helped by a sedative ANTIHISTAMINE medicine. Patches of eczema which become secondarily infected require antibiotic treatment. This is more likely to happen if scratching has occured.

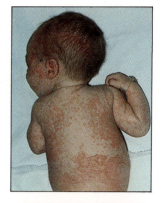

Cradle cap and seborrhoeic eczema A crusty brown greasy scalp found in young babies is known as cradle cap and may persist for some months after birth. In some babies there may be an associated rash, most marked in the nappy area, face and behind the ears. This is seborrhoeic eczema, which usually clears up during the first year.

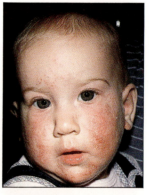

Atopic eczema Eczema may be red and inflamed, or dry and flaky. Both kinds of lesion are itchy, and can be made worse by scratching. It often starts on the face in babies, and there may be a family history of eczema, hay fever or asthma.

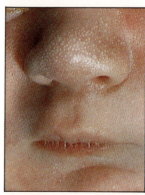

Milia Many new born babies have little white spots, principally on the nose and forehead. This is known as milia, and is a normal finding in newborns.

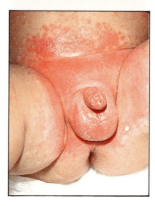

Nappy rash The skin of the nappy (diaper) area can become inflamed due to prolonged contact with urine. Frequent changing, and the use of a barrier cream is vital.

Children who have atopic eczema may develop asthma or hay fever at a later stage. These three conditions often occur in the same individual.

Nappy Rash

Nappy (diaper) rash, known as ammoniacal dermatitis, is due to contact of the skin with ammonia products in the urine. Initially there is a diffuse redness of lower addomen, genitalia and buttocks, in fact the whole area covered by a wet nappy. The folds and creases of skin may be spared. If more severe, the rash becomes moist and crusted and there may be some small ulcers where the skin surface has broken completely. Nappy rash is more likely to develop when the child has prolonged periods in wet nappies. Plastic pants, which prevent evaporation, can aggravate the rash. Changing nappies frequently, and using a barrier cream such as vaseline or zinc and castor oil over the nappy area, will largely prevent the rash. However, in most babies, a rash will develop from time to time.

To treat nappy rash, the whole nappy area should be kept clean and dry, with frequent changes of nappies, and with frequent washing of the skin to remove traces of urine. Exposure of the affected area leads to rapid healing but is not always practicable. If the rash has become infected, an antibiotic or antifungal cream may be helpful. The condition ceases to recur once the child is trained and out of nappies.

Keeping baby clean

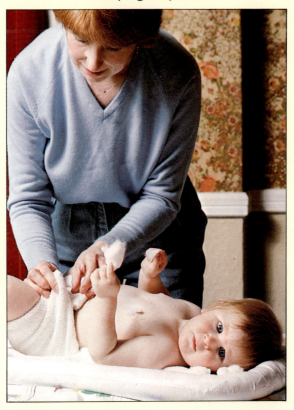
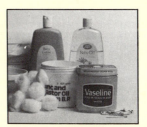

A baby does not have as much resistance to infection as an older child. Infections in early life are therefore serious and it is essential that you pay particular attention to keeping the baby clean. This includes frequent baths with regular washing of areas susceptible to infection, and prevention or treatment of nappy rash.

Bathing It is normal to bath a baby once a day after he is a week old, and as long as there is no complication or infection which would make it unadvisable. However, if you cannot keep up this routine all the time, you can at least wash the baby all over every day, paying particular attention to the nappy area and face.

The baby may not like being bathed at first, so be sure to hold him securely when giving him a bath. Cradle him in one arm and wash him carefully and gently with the other, but do this fairly quickly as a newborn baby will lose body heat rapidly and should not be in the bath for too long. As the baby gets older he will want to stay in the bath longer and will enjoy splashing around and playing with toys in the bath. **Never** leave a baby alone in the bath, not even for a minute, as he could easily drown.

Nappy rash is an inevitable condition at some stage of babyhood, particularly during teething or bouts of diarrhoea. The incidence of nappy rash can be greatly reduced by scrupulous care and hygiene when changing nappies.

It is imperative that nappies are changed frequently and that the nappy area is cleaned thoroughly at each nappy change. Disposable or terry towelling nappies can be used — it is a matter of preference.

The nappy area should be cleaned thoroughly with tissues or cotton wool, moistened with water, baby lotion or baby oil. Water can be drying to the skin, but some babies react to oils or lotions. After cleansing, the area should be dried thoroughly and if there is any sign of redness or irritation a barrier cream may be applied. For extensive nappy rash, exposure to the air is the most effective treatment, even if this is only convenient for short spells.

When washing terry nappies, first rinse and soak in an antiseptic solution for two to three hours, prior to washing. This will kill any germs. Use a very mild detergent and avoid fabric softeners as these can irritate a young baby's skin and exacerbate any existing nappy rash. Rinse the nappies thoroughly.

Other skin disorders

ALMOST ALL ADOLESCENTS develop some spots of acne on the face. Acne is a disorder of the sebaceous glands in the skin which normally produce a greasy secretion to keep the skin flexible and in good condition. In acne the sebaceous glands become blocked, so that the secretion is retained in the skin rather than being gradually released onto the surface. As a result the characteristic acne lesions develop, consisting of comedones or blackheads, red raised spots, and small pustules. If secondary infection occurs large angry looking pustules can develop.

Many factors contribute to the development of acne. Hormonal influences are obviously paramount, but diet, stress, and additional infection are also relevant. Acne is rare before the onset of puberty. It tends to be at its worst while the changes of puberty are taking place, gradually settles down thereafter, and is usually completely better by the late teens. Girls often find the skin is at its worst just before each period.

Some foods will make acne worse, and most dermatologists recommend restriction of the intake of chocolate, nuts and fizzy drinks. Acne often flares up when a young person is under stress.

There is, as yet, no treatment that is wholly effective in curing acne, and the aim is to try and limit the development of active lesions to prevent scarring. The skin should be well washed with soap twice daily, as this helps to degrease the skin and to prevent blockage of the sebaceous ducts in the skin surface. Ultraviolet light tends to improve the lesions, so exposure to sunlight is beneficial. Blackheads and pustules should not be squeezed, because this may damage the skin and encourage secondary infections, but a special extractor can be purchased and is effective in draining the sebaceous secretions. There are a variety of ointments which can be tried. None is of definite benefit for all patients.

In severe acne the doctor may recommend a prolonged antibiotic course to try and prevent the development of infected pustules. Permanent scarring as the result of acne only occurs in patients who have been severely affected, and is more likely if lesions become infected.

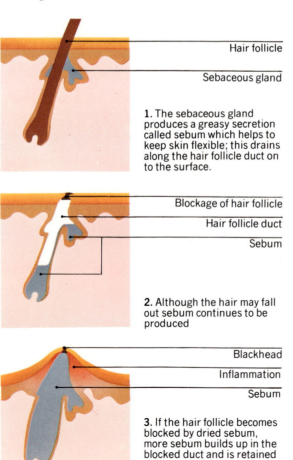

Hair follicle

Sebaceous gland

1. The sebaceous gland produces a greasy secretion called sebum which helps to keep skin flexible; this drains along the hair follicle duct on to the surface.

Blockage of hair follicle

Hair follicle duct

Sebum

2. Although the hair may fall out sebum continues to be produced

Blackhead

Inflammation

Sebum

3. If the hair follicle becomes blocked by dried sebum, more sebum builds up in the blocked duct and is retained in the skin. This causes a blackhead to form.

Treatment of Acne

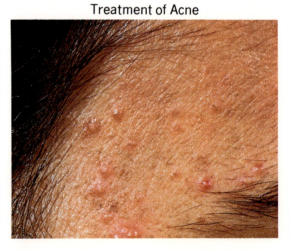

There is no treatment that is completely effective in curing acne. However certain measures can be taken to improve and control the condition and prevent scarring.

The skin should be well washed with a mild soap and hot water at least twice a day. Pimples, blackheads and whiteheads should not be squeezed as this can damage the skin and encourages secondary infection. Girls should use a minimum of cosmetics — greasy brands especially must be avoided. Chocolate and nuts should not be eaten. Ultraviolet light helps to dry the skin so adolescents with acne should be encouraged to be out in the sun as much as possible.

If acne is severe antibiotic treatment may be given for a long period. Reassurance and understanding is also essential as acne can be emotionally upsetting.

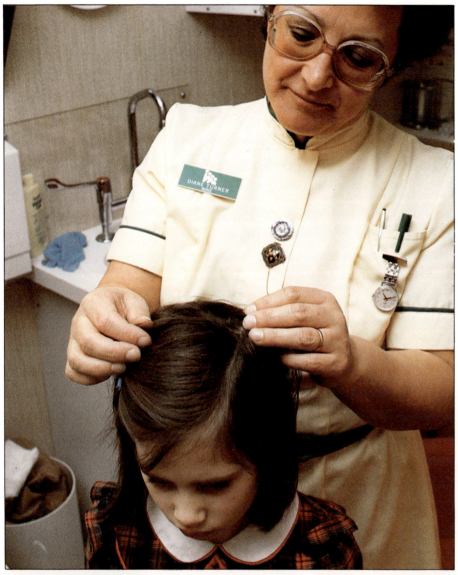

Head lice are often spread amongst children at school. They are tiny, but visible, insects that live on the scalp, sucking blood and injecting saliva. The eggs of lice (nits) are also visible. They look like tiny white grains in the hair. The nits of head lice cause intense itching. The skin can become infected with the repeated scratching and this results in swollen glands behind the ears.

If a child has lice the whole family should be checked and treated if necessary. Treatment is with a special insecticide shampoo or lotion which kills both insects and eggs. Clothes and bedclothes need thorough washing.

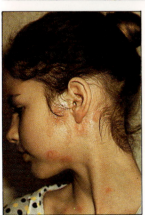

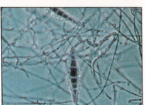

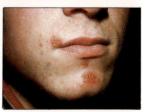

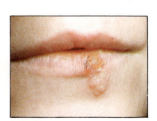

Ringworm (left) is a fungal infection of the skin or scalp. When the scalp is affected the hairs may break off leaving a bald patch. The causative fungus can be identified microscopically (above).

Impetigo is a contagious skin infection. It presents with crusty, bleeding spots over the face, trunk and limbs. Without treatment these spread rapidly. Treatment is with antibiotics and antibiotic creams.

Herpes simplex (cold sore) The familiar cold sores are due to a virus called herpex simplex which invades the skin and sometimes other areas. In some individuals attacks of herpes occur every time they get a cold.

The skeleton

THE SKELETON PROVIDES protection and support for the internal organs of the head, chest and abdomen. It also functions as an intricate and sophisticated series of levers which are moved by the muscles. Some idea of the complexity of the skeleton can be realized by considering the wide range of actions and activities of which we are capable — walking, running, sitting, holding, grasping, and many more. Each activity is carried out smoothly and harmoniously by the brain's control of the contraction and relaxation of the skeletal muscles which move the bones.

For protection, support, and leverage the bones need to be tough and rigid. They have a high mineral content with deposited calcium compounds as the main matrix, but this is reinforced with strong fibrous tissue. The outer part consists of compact bone, and in the middle the bone forms a lattice called trabecular bone. This structure gives strength to the frame, without being too heavy. Within this internal lattice is the bone marrow, where the red blood cells and many of the white blood cells are formed. Although strong and hard, bones consist of living tissue with a good blood supply and with bone cells situated in between the layers of deposited calcium salts. In the growing child the bones gradually

The skeleton The bones of the skeleton protect the internal organs and support the body. The bones of the limbs also act as levers moved by the muscles, to perform all physical activity.

Each bone has a hard outer layer, the cortex, and a trabeculated inner layer, the medulla. The bone consists of living cells between the bony supporting tissue, and needs a continuous blood supply to stay alive. In the gaps on the medullary bone are bone marrow cells producing blood cells for the circulation.

A cross-section through a long bone is enlarged to show its detail (below).

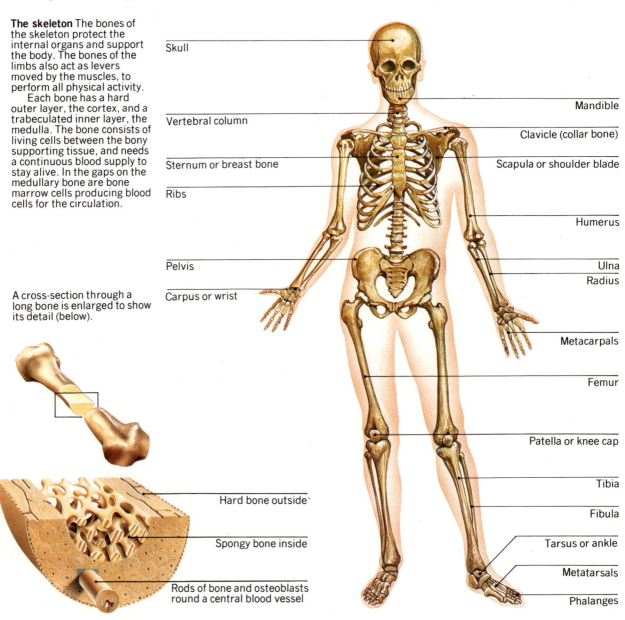

Skull

Vertebral column

Sternum or breast bone

Ribs

Pelvis

Carpus or wrist

Mandible

Clavicle (collar bone)

Scapula or shoulder blade

Humerus

Ulna

Radius

Metacarpals

Femur

Patella or knee cap

Tibia

Fibula

Tarsus or ankle

Metatarsals

Phalanges

Hard bone outside

Spongy bone inside

Rods of bone and osteoblasts round a central blood vessel

How bones grow

Growth of bones takes place throughout childhood. Cells called osteoblasts form the bones. The ends of the growing bones are composed of cartilage, and the osteoblasts gradually invade the cartilage and lay down new bone. In the foetus (right) only the shafts of the long bones have ossified (shown in red). Much of the bone is still cartilaginous.

Those joints where a lot of movement occurs are called synovial joints. Bones may also be joined by fibrous cartilage (for example between the vertebrae and the symphasis pubis) or, as in the skull, by bony fusion.

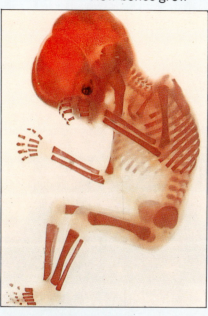

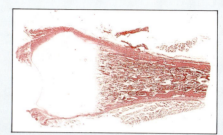

Microscopic section of growing bone

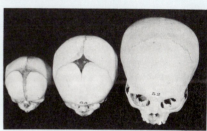

Gradual ossification of bones of the skull

change shape and are constantly being remodelled and strengthened to allow for growth and increased activity.

Growth of bones

At birth the bones of the skull are joined together to allow for growth; they fuse during childhood. Apart from most of the skull and the clavicles, the whole skeleton of the embryo is formed in cartilage which is gradually replaced by bone.

In childhood the ends of the long bones consist of cartilage, and it is here that growth takes place. This is caused by the deposition of calcium salts under the action of vitamin D. In rickets, where there is a deficiency of vitamin D, the ends of the bones do not develop and may become deformed.

In many growing bones the centre of the cartilage ossifies forming a separate piece of bone, the epiphysis which is joined to the shaft of the bone by the intervening cartilage. When the epiphysis fuses with the shaft, growth ceases.

Joint structure

The joints between bones which move together consist of smooth cartilage surfaces which are lubricated by fluid produced by the joint lining, the synovial fluid. The joint is surrounded by a fibrous capsule to give it strength and to hold the bones together, and there may be additional ligaments running between the bones to strengthen the joint.

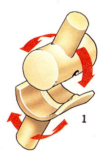

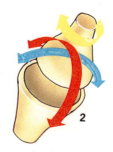

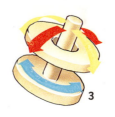

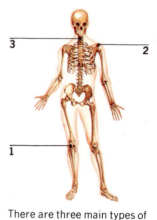

There are three main types of synovial joints —
1. **The hinge joint** which is found at the knee, elbow and fingers allows the joint to move in only one plane.
2. **The ball and socket joints**, found at the shoulder and hip, allow the long bones to move in several directions.
3. **The pivot joint**, between the first and second cervical vertebrae, enables rotation of the head as well as movement from side to side and front to back.

Fractures and dislocations

IF BONES ARE OVERTAXED they break, and this is known as a fracture. In childhood fractures are usually caused by falls, when running, climbing or tumbling downstairs, or by road accidents. If a child puts an arm out to save himself when he is falling, he may injure the arm or shoulder, and if he falls forcibly or awkwardly, he may break a leg.

Fractures in children do not always extend right across the bone, but may involve only one side. This is known as a greenstick fracture. If the skin is broken over the fracture it is termed open, and there is a risk of infection.

Fractures heal by new bone being formed gradually from either side of the break, to unite the two ends. The younger the child, the quicker this healing process will take place. The medical treatment of fractures consists first of the correction of any deformity present, and then immobilising it in a good position until healing has taken place.

A fracture may be suspected following a fall or injury because of pain, swelling, deformity of a bone or joint, or because of inability to use the limb. The child will need to be taken to an accident unit, and if the doctor suspects a fracture, Xrays are taken. These will reveal any break and show whether or not the bones are out of position. If there is deformity this will need to be corrected under an anaesthetic before the limb is immobilized in plaster. Not all fractures are treated in this manner. Leg injuries may need to be immobilized by traction, using weights attached to the leg, and collar bone fractures and some other arm injuries, may need to be treated with a special sling.

A plaster cast needs to be firm enough to give adequate suport, but not so tight that it interferes with the

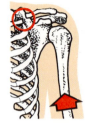

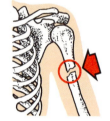

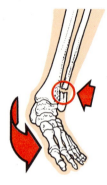

Collar bone fractures (top right) are usually due to indirect pressure such as a fall on the hand or on the shoulder. It is rare for them to happen from direct impact, instead the force is transmitted along the bone from the point of impact. A twisting fall or stumble (bottom right), can cause the ankle to bend excessively. Because of leverage tremendous pressure can be placed on the bone causing it to fracture.
A bone can be fractured directly at the point where the impact has taken place (middle right). For example, an arm could be hit by a moving object, such as a car.

A greenstick fracture is common in children because they have flexible, soft bones. The bone is partially broken on one side only.
A closed fracture is one where the skin is not broken over the bone. **A compond fracture** is where the surface of the skin has been penetrated so that the bone and surrounding tissue are exposed to infection. **A complicated fracture** (see inset) is where the blood vessels or organs adjacent to the bone are damaged by sharp bone fragments; this can occur in both compound and closed fractures. **A comminuted fracture** is where the bone is broken into several pieces.

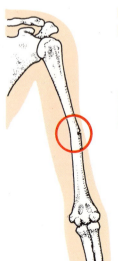

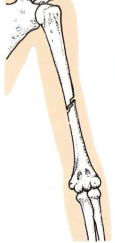

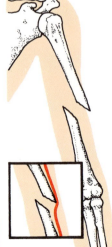

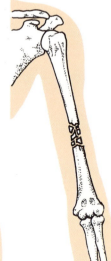

A greenstick fracture   A closed fracture   A compound fracture   A communited fracture

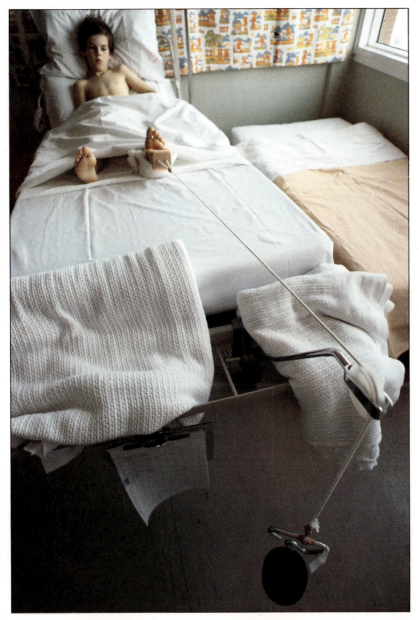

Traction enables broken bones to be pulled apart in order to get them or to keep them in the correct place. This is necessary when the muscles around the bone pull and contract and force the bone into an unsatisfactory position. Traction is used where it is not possible to hold the bones in place with a plaster or a splint.

Traction is applied by attaching weights to a child's limb either by means of adhesive tape or by placing a metal pin through a neighbouring bone.

Traction is also used to rest a limb when there is a suspected or definite bone disease, such as infection or arthritis.

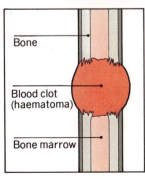

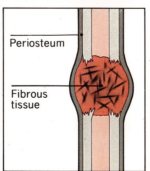

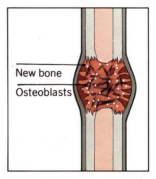

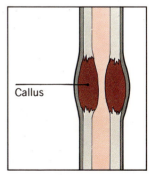

Bone Healing 1. When a bone breaks there is bleeding from the broken ends, giving rise to a collection of blood known as a haematoma.

2. This blood clots, and gradually fibrous tissue grows across it. The blood is gradually absorbed. Periosteum from around the outside of the bone grows round the haematoma to bridge the gap between the broken ends of bone.

3. Osteoblast cells, which form bone, grow out from the periosteum to lay down new bone around the fracture. This new bone is called callus.

4. When healing is complete the bone is joined as strongly as it was before. The callus gradually becomes smaller, and may disappear completely.

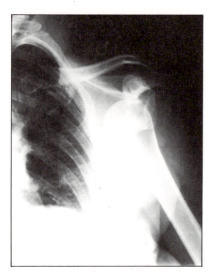

Dislocation of the shoulder The shoulder joint is very manoeuverable and as a result it can become dislocated fairly easily. When it is dislocated (see above and right) the two articular surfaces of the joint are forced out of position so that they are no longer in contact.

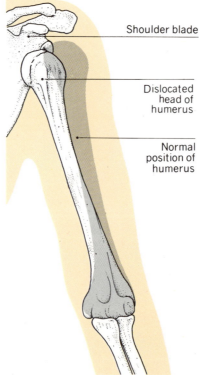

Shoulder blade

Dislocated head of humerus

Normal position of humerus

Congenital dislocation of the hip The hip, like the shoulder, is a ball and socket joint. The ball at the top of the thigh bone (femur) fits into the cup-shaped socket in the pelvis. In a dislocated hip joint the thigh bone is displaced and does not fit into the socket in the pelvis. Some babies are born with a dislocated hip or one that readily slips in and out of its socket.

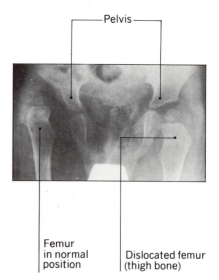

Pelvis

Femur in normal position

Dislocated femur (thigh bone)

circulation. If fingers and toes become swollen, blue, tingly, numb, or painful after a plaster has been applied, urgent medical aid should be sought. Immobilizing a fracture gives considerable pain relief, but in the early days after the injury analgesics may also be required. Soluble aspirin or paracetamol will usually suffice.

Common fractures in childhood

Falls on the oustretched hand in childhood may lead to fractures of the collar bone (clavicle), elbow or forearm, or the dislocation of the shoulder. Fractures involving the legs are less common, and usually involve road or riding accidents, or falling awkwardly when moving fast, as in football or skiing.

Skull fractures occur as a result of falls or accidents. They indicate that there was significant trauma to the head, and close observation is needed to determine whether there is any internal damage to brain or blood vessels. The actual break in the bone will heal without any special treatment.

Dislocations

A dislocation is the disruption of a joint so that the articular surfaces of the bones involved are no longer in contact. Usually dislocations arise as the result of injury. Shoulder and finger joints are the most prone to traumatic dislocation, but it can also occur at the elbow,

and less commonly at other joints. When a dislocation has occurred following an accident, the bones must be put back into place, reducing the dislocation, and then the joint must be supported until the capsule (casing of the joint) has healed. Sometimes operative reduction and repair is needed.

Congenital dislocation of the hip

Some babies are born with a looseness of the hip joint, so that the hip is either dislocated all the time, or readily slips in or out of its socket. If this is detected by routine examination in the newborn period it is relatively easy to correct by splinting for a few months. If not detected until the child begins to walk it will require operative treatment for correction. Congenital dislocation of the hip may run in families, so that if there is a family history babies should be examined carefully in the newborn period on more than one occasion.

Sprains

After an injury, a joint may be painful even though there has been no fracture or dislocation. The injury may have damaged the joint capsule or a ligament. Movements of the joint will be painful and there may be swelling. A firm bandage will usually be beneficial. *See pages 176-83 for first aid treatment of fractures, dislocations and sprains.*

Skeletal deformities

THE MOST COMMON skeletal disorders found in children are described below. If treatment is necessary, the child will generally be referred to an orthopaedic surgeon who specializes in correcting the deformities of children.

Bow legs and knock knees

Parents are often worried if their child does not have straight legs and instead the knees are bent inwards (knock knees) or outwards (bow legs). In children aged one to four years this is a fairly common anomaly, and providing there is no evidence of rickets or other bone diseases, no investigation or treatment is required. It is a developmental stage of growth, and the legs straighten as the child gets older.

Scoliosis

A scoliosis is a twisting deformity of the spine, so that there are curvatures from side to side as well as the natural curves backwards in the thoracic region and forwards in the lumbar region.

Scoliosis may result from a congenital defect of vertebral development or may be secondary to local disease of the spine. In some individuals scoliosis may be postural and can be fully corrected if the posture improves.

Talipes (Club feet)

Deformity of the ankle and foot, recognizable at birth, is known as talipes or club foot. There are two main types, with the foot bent either inwards or outwards. Early treatment with manipulation and strapping may be corrective. In more severe cases operative correction may be needed.

Intoeing (Metatarsus varus)

It is common to see turning in of the front of the foot in toddler-aged children. They may fall over more frequently than other children because their toes get intertwined, particularly on running. If the heel and the rest of the foot is normal, spontaneous improvement can be anticipated without treatment, and often the doctor will reassure the parents at the first consultation.

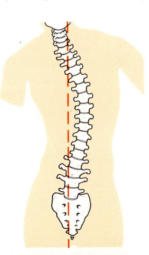

Scoliosis may also occur for unknown reasons at around the time of puberty. This is so-called idiopathic scoliosis and is more common in girls than boys. If untreated it may lead to unsightly and damaging deformity. If a teenager appears to be developing any assymetry of the spine or thorax, it should be assessed by an expert to see if any treatment is necessary. This diagram (right) shows the twisting of the vertebral column which occurs in scoliosis. The scoliosis in this boy was due to bad posture and was readily corrected (below right).

Fitting of shoes

When a child starts to walk there is real value in leaving him barefoot whenever conditions are suitable. This means that it is worth letting him go barefoot indoors until the age of two or three. When you do buy shoes for a child it is essential that they are comfortable. They should be big enough so that the toes are not cramped, but must not be so big that they almost fall off. Socks must also be large enough.

Small children outgrow their shoes very rapidly so it is worth parents checking regularly that shoes are large enough. Do not buy expensive shoes at this stage as fit is more important than quality.

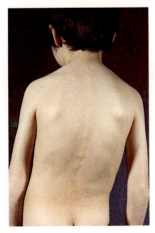

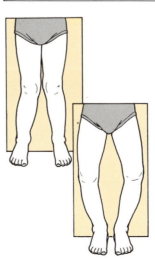

Bow legs and knock knees It is not uncommon for young children to have bow legs (bottom left) and knock knees (top left). The former are more obvious in the first two years of life, the latter tend to develop a little later. No treatment is usually necessary as these conditions disappear spontaneously.

A GUIDE TO MEDICAL TERMS

A large number of medical terms are derived from Latin and Greek. If you know the meaning of the Latin and Greek components, it will be easy to interpret many medical terms that at first sight seem complex. A selection is listed below. The position of the hyphen shows whether the component is placed at the beginning or the end of the term. In the United States the 'a' has been dropped from 'aemia' and 'haem'.

a-, an-: a lack of, an absence of
ab-: away from
ad-: towards, near to
-aemia: of the blood
andr-: of the male sex
anti-: against, opposing
-arch-, -arche-: first
arthr-: of a joint
audio-: of hearing, or sound
aut-, auto-: self
bi-: two
brady-: slowness
-cele: a swelling
-centesis: perforation
chron-: time
-cide: destroyer
contra-: against, opposite
cryo-: cold
-cyte: a cell
de-: removal, or loss
derm-: of the skin
dipl-: double
dys-: difficulty, abnormality
ec-, ect-: outside, external
-ectomy: surgical removal
em-, en-: inside, internal
end-: inner, within
enter-: of the intestine
epi-: upon, over
erythr-: red
ex-, exo-: outside of, outer
extra-: outside, beyond
fibr-: of fibrous tissue
-genic: producing
-gram: record, trace
-graph: a device that records

haem-: of the blood
hepat-: of the liver
hetero-: dissimilar
hemeo-: alike
hydr-: of water, or fluid
hyp-, hypo-: deficiency in, lack of
hyper-: excess of
-iasis: a disease state
inter-: between
intra-: inside
-itis: inflammation
laparo-: of the abdomen or loins
leuc-, leuk-: white
-lysis: breaking up
macro-: large
mal-: disorder, abnormality
-mania: compulsion, obsession
mast-: of the breast
megal-: abnormally large
-megaly: abnormal enlargement
mes-: middle
met-, meta-: a) change, e.g. metabolism; b) distant, e.g. metastasis
micro-: small
myo-, my-: of the muscles
myelo-: of the spine
nephr-: of the kidneys
neur-: of the nerves
-oma: a tumor
-osis: a disease state
ost-: of bone
-otomy: a surgical examination

pan-: all
para-: a) near, e.g. paramedian; b) like, e.g. paratyphoid; c) abnormal, e.g. paraesthesia
path-: of disease
-pathy: disease
-penia: deficiency
peri-: near, around
-philia: craving, love for
phleb-: of the veins
-plasia: formation
-phlegia: paralysis
pneo-: of respiration
-poiesis: formation
poly-: many
pre-: a) before, e.g. prenatal; b) in front of, e.g. prevertebral
pro-: before, in front of
proct-: of the anus and rectum
rhin-: of the nose
-stasis: standing still
sub-: below
tox-: poisonous
trans-: through, across
-trophy: growth, development
vas-: a vessel

Section Three:
Glossary

The glossary provides the reader
with information on rare diseases and
conditions which are not covered
in the text.
It also gives some further
explanation of information referred to in
other sections of the book.

ABSCESS
An abscess is a cavity containing pus, a result of infection by bacteria. The body mounts a defence against the bacteria and large numbers of white blood cells move into the affected area, causing inflammation. Pus is a mixture of bacteria, inflammatory cells and body fluid. Abscesses can occur anywhere in the body where there is infection.

ACHONDROPLASIA
Achondroplasia is one form of short-limbed short stature. Specific diagnosis is not always easy, but may be important as some forms of this disorder are genetic. Achondroplasia is associated with short, but strong, arms and legs with a fairly short body and a slightly protruding forehead.

ADOPTION
Adoptions are normally arranged through an adoption agency or through a social service department. The child's interests are paramount when arranging the adoption. Social and perhaps medical reports will be obtained on the prospective adoptive parents before placement, and a trial period will be needed before the adoption can be legally finalized. Before the child is placed for adoption a medical examination is needed, and any abnormality will be reported to the new parents.

ADRENAL GLANDS
The adrenal glands are two small organs situated on top of the kidneys. They produce adrenalin and other hormones which are essential for life. The hormones are involved in the control of blood pressure, water and salt balance, and carbohydrate and protein turnover in the body.

Androgens which are essential for normal male development are also released. If the adrenal glands are abnormal or are removed, replacement therapy with steroids can be given.

ALOPECIA
Alopecia is the loss of hair. The common causes in children include emotional disturbance, ringworm of the scalp, and drug or radiation treatment given for leukaemia or brain tumours. In none of these conditions is the hair loss permanent, but psychiatric help may be necessary if the emotional disturbance is severe. Ringworm can be treated appropriately. Wigs are available for those whose hair has fallen out if the loss is extensive.

AMNIOCENTESIS
Amniocentesis is the process by which a specimen of amniotic fluid is taken with a needle in order to examine the condition of the foetus in the womb.

ANAESTHETIC
An anaesthetic is a drug which temporarily abolishes sensation. General anaesthetics also send the patient to sleep, and are mostly administered by inhalation, but some may be given intravenously. Local anaesthetics inhibit the function of nerves in a restricted area.

ANALGESICS
Analgesics are pain killing drugs. Aspirin and paracetamol ('Calpol' in syrup form) are the two most frequently given to children. Both are fever-reducing drugs and a high dosage of aspirin has an anti-inflammatory effect, making it useful in the treatment of arthritis.

Children need stronger analgesics only after operations or major accidents.

ANTIBIOTICS
Antibiotics are drugs which kill bacteria, or stop their growth. Although they are usually given in short courses by mouth or injection, they can also be used safely to give long term protection (prophylaxis) to children with recurrent infections. The most common example of this latter use is in the prevention of recurrent urinary tract infections.

ANTICONVULSANT DRUGS
Anticonvulsants are drugs which prevent or terminate convulsions. They are given in doses sufficient to achieve a 'therapeutic level' in the blood. This is the level which prevents fits without causing side-effects. If this level is achieved and maintained, most fits are controlled with one drug, but a few epileptics need a combination of drugs prescribed by a specialist. To be effective, the drugs must be taken regularly; sudden omission can cause a recurrence of the fits. Doctors normally carry a quick-acting anticonvulsant which can be injected to stop a fit once it has started.

APHASIA
Aphasia is the absence or loss of the ability to express oneself by speech or writing, or the absence or loss of the ability to understand the same. Delayed onset of speech in children calls for careful assessment of the child and his family, with particular reference to the child's general development and hearing. Children with aphasia may need help from an audiologist, a speech therapist or a psychiatrist, depending on the cause of the aphasia.

ARTHRITIS
Arthritis is inflammation of the joints and the tissues around

them. In children the most common types are rheumatoid arthritis (Still's disease), septic arthritis, and transient arthritis and synovitis (inflammation of the joint linings) after trauma or certain viral and bacterial infections. Affected joints are hot, painful and swollen.

In septic arthritis the patient is ill, with a high fever and poor appetite in addition to the specific joint problems. Bed rest, antibiotics and possibly surgery to drain the infection, are the essential components of treatment.

Rheumatoid arthritis can be present from infancy onwards. Initial symptoms may be a fever, general malaise and a rash, with later involvement of the joints. There may also be an inflammation of the front of the eye in some forms of the disease. Treatment is with anti-inflammatory drugs, such as aspirin, and PHYSIOTHERAPY when necessary. In a few cases other drugs may be indicated. The prognosis varies according to the form the disease takes, but on the whole it tends to 'burn itself out' in more than three-quarters of affected children, who then go on to lead normal lives.

ATOPY
Atopy is the name applied to the spectrum of related conditions, eczema, asthma and hay fever. There appears to be an inherited disposition to atopic disease, but environmental factors are also important.

AUTISM
Autism is an uncommon mental illness starting in infancy. The child seems to live in a world of his own, avoiding eye to eye contact, disliking cuddles or other warm approaches, and does not relate to the outside world by

speech. Often repetitive movements or habits develop. Although some autistic children achieve a degree of recovery, the illness usually lasts into adult life.

BILIARY ATRESIA
Biliary atresia is a congenital absence of bile ducts. As a result bile cannot drain from the liver and jaundice develops within a week of birth, and persists. The condition must be distinguished from neonatal hepatitis. When the atresia affects the ducts outside the liver, surgical treatment is possible if an early diagnosis is made. Intrahepatic biliary atresia cannot be treated and the child normally dies from liver failure in early childhood.

BLOOD GROUPS
There are two main ways of grouping blood, according to the markers which are present on the surface of the red blood cells. The ABO system refers to four possible groups so that a person belongs to either an 'A' group, a 'B' group, an 'AB' group or an 'O' group. The other system involves the rhesus factor in the blood. Eighty five per cent of people are rhesus (Rh) positive, while only fifteen per cent have no rhesus factor and are classified as rhesus (Rh) negative. If a transfusion is necessary, the blood must be compatible and therefore it is cross-matched to check that there will be no reaction during the transfusion.

Some serious illnesses of newborn babies are due to their being a different rhesus group from their mothers. See RHESUS INCOMPATIBILITY.

BLOOD IN THE STOOLS
The most common cause of passing blood with a stool is a minor abrasion or tear in the anal mucosa or skin. This will bleed a

little as a large, hard stool is passed and blood can be seen on the surface of the stool. Passing such a stool is painful and the child may become reluctant to defaecate and subsequently become constipated, causing further pain. Regular toilet habits and a diet designed to soften stools will help, but sometimes medication may be necessary. If constipation is severe it can cause a deeper split in the anal canal, known as an ANAL FISSURE. This condition may require a small surgical operation.

If red blood is mixed into the stool, and particularly if it is accompanied by mucus, inflammation or infection of the bowel may be present. Red blood alone may indicate bleeding from the lower bowel, from a polyp (a harmless tumour), or from a diverticulum (bulge in the large intestine), or it may be due to a blood disorder. Bleeding from higher up the bowel results in the partial digestion of the blood which is then passed as a black tarry stool (melaena). Whatever the cause of the bleeding a medical opinion should be sought.

BLOOD IN THE VOMIT
Blood is seen in vomit of children who have been retching forcefully and repeatedly. If a few fine blood vessels rupture around the top of the stomach it is seldom serious. Swallowed blood, usually after a nose bleed or dental extraction, is often vomited. The vomiting of large amounts of fresh red blood is very rare in children. Medical advice should be sought immediately if this occurs.

BOILS
Boils are abscesses in the skin. They are caused by staphylococcal bacteria and may

153

enter a dirty cut or graze. However some children develop recurrent boils, and they may be carrying the infection in their noses as well as on the skin. Recurrent boils tend to occur when the child is 'run down' after a severe viral infection, or from hard work and worry. In these circumstances a long course of antibiotics and a nasal cream will break the cycle of infection, and a period of rest will be beneficial.

BONE MARROW
The marrow is the soft central part of the bone. Blood cells are made there and released into the circulation. Examination of the marrow is important in blood diseases such as leukaemia and severe anaemia. A sample can be taken from the top of the hip bone or other sites and examined under the microscope to reveal the numbers and types of cell present.

Bone marrow transplant is sometimes used in the treatment of leukaemia and certain rare disorders affecting the marrow. The recipient's marrow is killed off by a heavy course of irradiation, and donor cells injected into the circulation. If the transplant is successful, they settle into the recipient's marrow space and grow there.

BRAIN TUMOURS
Brain tumours in children cause vomiting and headaches, which are worse in the morning after waking. Unsteadiness (ataxia) irritability and lethargy may develop later but convulsions are very rare. In children under five, enlargement of the head may occur. Different types of brain tumour start in slightly different ways depending on the age of the child, but most of them spread malignantly through the brain. Complete surgical removal is not

always possible. Treatment is a combination of partial surgical removal, radiation and drug therapy. The prognosis depends upon the type and site of the tumour. Certain less common tumours can be completely excised, and the child cured. The more common medulloblastoma, when treated as above, can now be cured in up to 50 per cent of cases. Even when a cure is impossible, treatment to suppress symptoms (palliation) can frequently be achieved and, with the relief of symptoms, the child and his family can enjoy months or years of life together.

BREAST ENLARGEMENT
Babies of both sexes have breast tissue and under the influence of maternal hormones, the breasts enlarge prior to delivery. After birth a little milk may be discharged from the nipples. No treatment is necessary, and the breasts soon become smaller and stop secreting milk once the withdrawal from the influence of maternal hormones is complete.

More rarely the breast may be infected soon after birth. The baby is irritable, feverish and lethargic. The affected breast becomes hot, inflamed and tender and treatment with antibiotics is needed.

BRONCHODILATORS
Bronchodilators are drugs used in the treatment of asthma. Their action is to open up (dilate) the constricted airways (bronchi and bronchioles) which cause the wheezing and shortness of breath from which asthmatics suffer. They can be inhaled or taken by mouth, using a spray or special inhaler which releases a fine powder capsule. Younger children can also be given specially designed inhalers for use both in the home and in hospital.

CATARACTS
Cataracts are opacities in the lens of the eye. They are very rare in children who are otherwise healthy, but occur in babies whose mothers had German measles (rubella) early in pregnancy, and in certain rare metabolic disorders. Most congenital cataracts should be removed within two months of birth. Contact lenses are then worn to overcome the refractive error caused by the loss of the eye lens.

CATARRH
Catarrh is the profuse nasal discharge which accompanies a cold. If a catarrhal discharge persists after the cold has apparently cleared, sinusitis should be suspected. This may cause a troublesome cough at night soon after the child lies down, when the catarrh runs backwards down the nose and irritates the back of the throat. This is known as a post-nasal drip.

CATHETER
A catheter is the special name for any hollow tube inserted into the body. Catheters can be used for draining the bladder, to give infusions into a vein or artery, or even passed along a blood vessel into the heart for special investigations.

CHILD ABUSE
Child abuse may take the form of non-accidental injury to children (the 'battered baby'), or less obvious forms such as poisoning, sexual assault, physical neglect and emotional deprivation. It occurs in all levels of society, and one particular child may be abused within an otherwise 'normal' family. Once the diagnosis has been made, it should be recognized that both

parents and child need help. The parents themselves may have had a deprived childhood. With support, and possibly with the relief of other stresses within the family, whether financial, marital or psychological, many families remain united and the parents continue to care for their children.

When the abuse is severe, the child may have to be removed from the family. A placement which is best for the child is the main consideration in these circumstances. Many children can be returned to their parents under supervision once things have calmed down.

CHILD GUIDANCE CLINICS

Difficult children who do not settle satisfactorily into school life may be referred to a clinic, which is staffed by a child psychiatrist, a psychologist and psychiatric social worker. Usually the child and his parents are seen together and separately, and a rational approach to the management of the child's behaviour or other problems is offered. Initial referral is often by the school, but the clinic can be approached directly by parents through the school or local education authority.

CHROMOSOMES

Chromosomes are microscopic strands which are present within the nucleus of every cell. They carry the genes which determine the inherited characteristics of the individual. Normal children have 46 chromosomes, arranged in pairs. One from each pair is derived from the mother, and one from the father. One pair of chromosomes is known as the sex chromosomes as they determine the sex of the individual. If both are the same (called XX) the child is female, and if different (called

XY) the child is male.

Abnormal numbers or forms of chromosomes occur in certain diseases (eg. Down's syndrome, Turner's syndrome).

COELIAC DISEASE

Coeliac disease is caused by sensitivity to gluten, a protein found in wheat and other cereals, and as a result the lining of the small bowel fails to digest and absorb food normally. The classic onset of coeliac disease is when the child fails to thrive soon after being weaned onto a full diet, develops mild diarrhoea and a distended abdomen and is rather subdued and miserable. Frequently the onset is insidious and the diagnosis may not be made for years, even into adulthood.

Diagnosis is confirmed by a jejunal biopsy. In this procedure the child is sedated and a small capsule is attached to a fine tube to which suction is applied. A small piece of the lining of the bowel is sucked into the capsule and cut off and this is examined under a microscope.

Coeliac disease is treated with a 'gluten-free' diet which excludes protein from the bowel. As the sensitivity is always present, this diet must be followed throughout life. Usually a second biopsy is performed some years after the initial diagnosis to confirm that the correct diagnosis was made.

COLD SORES

Cold sores are the painful spots which occur at the corners of the mouth during a cold or upper respiratory tract infection. They are caused by a herpes virus and tend to flare up with each new cold. In between attacks the virus lives silently in the tissues. Local treatment with moisturising cream gives some relief. The application of an ice pack also helps.

COLOSTRUM

For the first few days after birth the breasts secrete a clear fluid called colostrum, before milk production is established. Colostrum helps to protect the newborn baby from infection.

CLEFT PALATE

Cleft palate occurs alone or with a hare lip. The cleft extends from the soft palate forwards and exposes both nasal cavities. The immediate problems are those of feeding, especially when the lip is involved. Breast feeding can be difficult but not impossible, and special teats are available to help both breast and bottle feeding. Surgical repair of the palate is usually at about one year and, following this the palate is ready for normal speech to develop.

COLIC

Colic is an acute abdominal pain which waxes and wanes in intensity. It may originate in the bowel, the renal tract or the bile ducts of the liver. The only type of colic common in children is intestinal; the others will not be considered here. The 'three months' or 'evening' colic occurs late in the day in babies up to three months of age, although in some it persists for longer. A typical attack starts with the baby suddenly starting to scream, pulling the legs up and going red in the face. It may last for a few minutes only, or for half an hour. As the attack abates, the baby sobs pitifully and either falls asleep or suffers a recurrence of the pain. Wind, tension in the baby, tension in the mother, milk allergies, maternal diet (in breast-fed babies) and poor feeding techniques have all been suggested as possible causes of intestinal colic. Any mother with a screaming baby is bound to be worried, but this type of colic passes off within the first half of infancy, the babies suffer no permanent physical harm and do not appear different from other children as they grow older. Each mother may find a particular 'trick' to help her own baby until spontaneous recovery occurs. Some babies appear to be helped by medication given in liquid form which alters the mobility of the bowel.

Colic in an older infant or child may have a different significance. If the child is ill, pale and vomiting in addition to having colic, possible diagnoses include blockage of the intestine, gastroenteritis or appendicits. It may also be due to a transient minor disturbance of the bowels, so it is important that colic in an older child is viewed in the light of his general condition. Medical help should be sought if the colic is severe and persistent, or if the child is ill in other ways.

CONJUNCTIVITIS

Conjuctivitis is an inflammation of the lining of the eyelids and the front of the eyes. It can be caused by infection, allergy, chemicals or exposure to dry, dusty winds. The eye feels sore and gritty. It weeps and may discharge pus. Infectious conjunctivitis should be treated with antibiotic ointments or drops. Some episodes are viral in origin, and although ointments may then provide symptomatic relief and prevent secondary infection, the eye eventually heals itself. Allergic conjunctivitis can occur as part of hay fever, or in isolation. Persistent or seasonal symptoms merit a consideration of allergy as the cause of the problem.

Treatment is with drops which damp down the allergic response, and the allergen itself should be avoided if practicable. See also STICKY EYE.

CROHN'S DISEASE

Crohn's disease is a chronic relapsing inflammatory disease of the bowel. Characteristically the patches of inflammation occur in different places at different times. Although lesions may occur anywhere between mouth and anus, the disease is one which usually affects the end of the small bowel. The child experiences pain, loss of appetite and an altered bowel movement.

CYST

A cyst is an abnormal fluid-filled swelling. In childhood cysts occasionally occur as remnants of structures which exist in embryonic life, but they later disappear.

CYSTIC FIBROSIS

Cystic fibrosis affects the lungs and digestive system. The mucous secretions of the lungs and pancreas are thick and sticky, and these organs fail to function properly. The lungs retain sputum, and are slowly damaged by recurrent infections which are slow to clear. The digestive functions of the pancreas are affected, food is not absorbed properly and weight gain tends to be poor. Some babies with cystic fibrosis have a thick sticky stool in their bowel at birth; this may have to be removed surgically.

Treatment consists of physiotherapy to the lungs, and antiobiotics for infections. Pancreatic enzymes are taken in capsules to compensate for the deficiency in digestion. Many children with cystic fibrosis now live a full life well into adulthood, but childhood deaths still occur in those more severely affected.

Cystic fibrosis is a recessively inherited disorder. Both parents of an affected child are unaffected carriers of the disease. If they have had one child with cystic fibrosis, there is a one in four chance that each of their future children will be affected. Current research includes attempts to develop a reliable test for antenatal diagnosis; progress is being made and such a test may soon be established.

DIABETES INSIPIDUS

Disease of part of the pituitary gland may cause a deficiency of a hormone, which leads to the production of large amounts of urine, and consequent excessive thirst, a condition known as diabetes insipidus. It should not be confused with the more common condition of diabetes mellitus *(see page 94)*. Diabetes insipidus can be treated with natural or synthetic hormone replacement.

DIALYSIS

Dialysis is the artificial 'washing' of the blood in children with kidney failure. In haemodialysis, blood is circulated through a 'kidney machine' which removes waste products before returning the blood to the body. In peritoneal dialysis, fluid is flushed in and out of the peritoneal cavity in the abdomen through a small plastic tube inserted into the front of the abdomen. While the fluid is in the cavity, it absorbs the waste products normally excreted by the kidney.

DIPHTHERIA

Diphtheria is an acute infection of the throat. It is now rare in this country as a result of improved hygiene, living conditions generally and immunization in infancy. The symptoms are fever, headache, general malaise and a sore throat. Spots appear on the tonsils and spread to form a continuous membrane over the back of the throat.

Diphtheria toxoid is part of the

triple vaccine given in infancy or it can be given alone, or with tetanus toxoid.

DUODENUM

The duodenum is the first part of the small intestine. It runs from the pyloric end of the stomach to the jejunum, the second part of the small intestine. The duodenum curves round the pancreas, and receives the pancreatic duct and the common bile duct from the liver.

ENZYMES

Enzymes are proteins produced in the body which facilitate the different chemical reactions of the body. For example the breakdown of food into constituent nutrients is performed by the reactions of digestive enzymes, while other enzymes control aspects of metabolism such as respiration and excretion.

FISTULA

An abnormal connection between two hollow organs, or between a hollow organ and the skin. A tracheo-oesophageal fistula is a congenital connection between the windpipe and gullet. Other fistulae are acquired as the result of infection, trauma or other disease.

FORESKIN (PREPUCE)

In infants the foreskin is often attached underneath the tip of the penis and it should not be pulled back forcibly, as pain, bleeding, and swelling of the penis will result.

Ninety per cent of those foreskins not retractable at birth become so by the age of two. If the foreskin becomes inflamed, frequent baths are a comfort and an aid to healing, but sometimes an antibiotic is needed. See also CIRCUMCISION page 110.

GLUE SNIFFING

Inhalation of the vapours of glues, solvents and polishes which induces a feeling of euphoria. The chemicals so inhaled are toxic, and long-term damage to the brain can occur. Tell-tale signs are a deterioration in concentration and school performance, confusion, sleepiness and loss of recent memory. There may be a rash around the mouth, the smell of glue and spots of it on clothes.

GROWING PAINS

Growing pains occur in approximately four per cent of schoolchildren, most commonly between six and thirteen years of age. There are pains in the calves or thighs at night, often described as 'aching' or 'heavy', and pain may occur in other limbs. They are not associated with disease, and settle down spontaneously. Despite the general acceptance of the name, the pains are not caused by growth, but the name is perpetuated as doctors tend to use the term in a reassuring way to indicate the benign nature of the symptoms to parents.

HAEMOPHILIA

Haemophilia is an inherited disorder of the blood which only affects boys. It presents in the second half of infancy with excessive bruising and prolonged bleeding during teething or after superficial cuts. Later, spontaneous bleeding into joints and muscles is frequent in the most severely affected. Treatment is with an infusion of plasma concentrates to replace the missing clotting factor.

HALITOSIS (bad breath)

Halitosis in children is unusual. It is caused by poor oral and dental hygiene, severe tonsillitis and some pneumonias which produce an offensive sputum. A foreign body in the nose may cause bad breath. The cause of minor halitosis is seldom found and mildly offensive breath is usually not associated with illness.

HARE LIP

Hare lip is the split in the lip which can occur in association with cleft palate. If it is severe the lip is pushed forward and the cleft extends into the nostril. Surgical correction is usually within three months of birth; cosmetic results are excellent.
(See also page 45)

HEALTH VISITOR

Health visitors are registered nurses attached to general practices who have had further training in the health, growth and development of children. Their role is principally supportive and preventive, offering guidance on growth, feeding and diet, immunization and developmental screening.

HENOCH SCHÖNLEIN PURPURA (Anaphylactoid purpura)

Henoch Schönlein purpura is a disease which most commonly presents with a blotchy red rash on the legs and buttocks as a result of blood leaking out of damaged capillaries. Abdominal pain can occur when similar lesions appear in the bowel and there may be associated bleeding. There may also be a transient arthritis.

Inflammation of the kidneys (nephritis) also occurs and very occasionally leads on to chronic kidney failure. Usually the disease lasts only a few weeks, and the child is not unduly ill. It is a result of abnormal immune reactions, but the exact cause is not yet established.

HYDROCEPHALUS
Hydrocephalus is an increase in the size of the fluid-filled ventricles in the centre of the brain. This arises either when there is a blockage of the flow of cerebro-spinal fluid away from the ventricles, or when there is over-production or under-absorption of the fluid. As the fluid accumulates, the head grows rapidly and in young children the bones separate. Hyrdocephalus occurs in association with spina bifida and other malformations of the central nervous system. It can also develop after meningitis, after haemorrhages in the ventricles of premature babies, or with a brain tumour. Hydrocephalus is relieved by draining the ventricles through a plastic tube and valve system which ends in the chest or abdomen.

HYPOSPADIAS
Hypospadias is the condition in which the urethra (the tube from the bladder to the tip of the penis) opens onto the under-surface of the penis. It occurs in approximately one in 350 males and varies in severity from a mild deformity, where the urethra opens a few millimetres below and behind the tip, to a more complex situation, in which the opening is on the perineum or scrotum. Many boys have such a mild degree of hypospadias that surgery is unnecessary. Where correction is indicated, most will need just one operation in the first two years; in more severe forms two procedures may be necessary, but surgery is usually completed by the age of four.

INTERNAL BLEEDING
This is potentially dangerous because a large volume of blood may be lost from the circulation before any injury is apparent. A ruptured liver or spleen after a severe blow to the abdomen are the commonest causes of silent internal bleeding. Although not truly 'internal' a fractured femur in a child bleeds heavily into the thigh.

INTESTINAL WORMS
Threadworms are common in children, but the majority of infections are asymptomatic. The only symptom of which the child is likely to complain is itchiness around the bottom, particularly at night. The thin short white worms are seldom seen. Treatment has to be for the whole family: two doses of medicine at fortnightly intervals will cure the infection.

Roundworms are pale and slightly larger than an earthworm. They may be vomited or even passed with a stool. Most sufferers are asymptomatic, but occasionally colic or even obstruction of the bowel occurs. The larvae migrate through the lungs and cause a cough and brief respiratory illness. Roundworms are rare in developed countries except where families are living without adequate toilet facilities.

INTUSSUSCEPTION
Intussusception occurs when a segment of bowel is pulled down the centre of the bowel causing a blockage of the intestine. This leads to attacks of colic, vomiting and sometimes the passing of a bloody stool. It is most common in the first two years, but can occur up to the age of six. It is diagnosed by clinical examination and *barium enema Xray* examination. In most cases, once the barium study has confirmed the diagnosis, a little pressure is applied to the barium in the bowel. This pushes the intussuscepted bowel back into place. When this fails, or if the procedure is contraindicted because of the child's poor state of health, surgery is necessary.

INVOLUNTARY MOVEMENTS
Involuntary movements can be divided into four main types. **TICS** are involuntary repetitious grimaces, usually just of the face, but occasionally of the trunk and limbs. They are almost always indicative of tension and anxiety in the child. Parents should not scold the child or try to repress the tics directly. Many tics disappear if the child is relieved of his worries and anxieties. Psychiatric help may be needed if the attacks persist. **TREMOR** is a fine quivering, most easily seen in the hands. It occurs with anxiety and fear. Fine tremor is present in thyrotoxicosis (overactivity of the thyroid gland). A coarse, flapping tremor is seen in serious liver disease. Intention tremor occurs in children with cerebellar disease, and worsens as the child gets closer to the object he wishes to touch or pick up. **CHOREA** is an irregular jerking movement which is now very rare. One form of chorea used to be a complication of rheumatic fever. **ATHETOSIS** is a sinuous writhing movement seen in some children with cerebral palsy.

JEJUNUM
The middle part of the small intestine, between the duodenum and the ileum.

KIDNEY FAILURE
Causes of kidney failure in childhood include congenital malformations of the kidney and renal tract, chronic undetected urinary tract infections with reflux of urine back to the kidney, and specific types of renal

damage in the immune processes which occur after certain diseases. The child with renal failure has general malaise, poor appetite, failure to thrive and lethargy. Later on, hypertension, coma and fits may develop. Treatment may include relief of any obstructions to the flow of urine, special diets and medication. Dialysis and transplants are needed for those with terminal kidney failure.

KIDNEY TRANSPLANT
A child who suffers terminal kidney failure can survive only with dialysis or with a kidney transplant. At present the three year survival after transplantation with a tissue-matched kidney is approximately seventy five per cent. The transplanted organ is protected from rejection by drugs which suppress the body's immune responses. If a first transplant fails, dialysis can be resumed, or a further transplant undertaken.

LABYRINTH
A name sometimes given to the structures of the inner ear, the semicircular canals and cochlea. They are embedded in bone and early anatomists noted the resemblance to caves in a rock, and gave the name labyrinth.

LEAD POISONING
This was more common when lead was used for water pipes and household paints. Chronic ingestion of lead results in general malaise, abdominal pains, anaemia and, in severe cases, coma. Such severe poisoning is now rarely seen. It has been found that urban children have higher blood lead levels than children living in the country. This is because of more prolonged exposure to petrol fumes which contain lead. There is some evidence that this slight increase,

whilst not causing overt lead poisoning, may have a harmful effect upon intelligence and performance of urban children.

MECONIUM
Meconium is the greenish sticky faecal contents of the newborn infant. The meconium is normally passed within a few hours of birth.

MESENTERY
The small intestine is attached to the posterior wall of the abdominal cavity by a membrane called the mesentery. It contains arteries, veins, and lymphatic vessels going to and from the intestine.

MENINGES
The membranes on the outside of the brain which give support and protection are known as the meninges. There are three layers of the meninges, the dura mater, the arachnoid and the pia mater. Meningitis is an infection of the meninges.

MENINGITIS
Meningitis is an infection of the meninges, the protective layers adjacent to and surrounding the brain and spinal cord. The symptoms are headache, photophobia, stiff neck and fever. The diagnosis is confirmed by a lumbar puncture, which is the insertion of a thin needle between the lower lumbar vertebrae to remove a sample of cerebro-spinal fluid for laboratory examination. Examination of this fluid reveals whether the meningitis has been caused by viruses or by bacteria, including tuberculosis. Viral meningitis needs only symptomatic treatment; complete recovery occurs within a few days. Bacterial meningitis can be more serious, and is treated with a

course of antibiotics which are usually given intravenously at first. Tuberculous meningitis is only occasionally seen. Most children recover completely from bacterial meningitis, but a few, particularly those in whom the diagnosis and treatment is delayed, may develop a degree of deafness. HYDROCEPHALUS may also develop in babies.

MICROCEPHALY
Microcephaly is a head which is disproportionately small for the age and body size of a child. Poor head growth is usually the result of poor brain growth. Although head size is not an absolute indicator of intelligence, almost all microcephalic children are handicapped. Causes include congenital infections (e.g. rubella), malformations of the brain, and damage from a lack of oxygen in the perinatal period.

MUSCULAR DYSTROPHY
The muscular dystrophies are a group of diseases in which the muscles degenerate and weaken. The symptoms, age of onset and rate of progression vary from one type of dystrophy to another. Muscular dystrophies are inherited diseases, but many new cases occur without a preceding family history. Duchenne muscular dystrophy, which only affects boys, is the commonest form in childhood. By three or four years the sufferers walk slowly, cannot climb stairs and fall frequently. By the age of ten they are confined to a wheelchair and die from chest infections and general debility in their late teens or early twenties. There are other less severe forms of muscular dystrophy which progress more slowly.

NEPHRITIS
Nephritis is an inflammation of

the kidney with a loss of protein and sometimes blood in the urine. The kidney may not function normally and the blood pressure may rise. The damage to the kidney is a result of altered or abnormal immune reactions within the body.

NEPHROTIC SYNDROME
Nephrotic syndrome is the result of a nephritis which results in heavy protein loss in the urine. As a result of this and other disturbances in protein metabolism, the protein levels in the blood fall, fluid retention occurs and the patient becomes swollen (oedematous). In young children the condition usually responds well to steroid therapy. Relapses may occur when the steriods are withdrawn, and repeated courses have to be given.

NEUROBLASTOMA
Neuroblastomas are highly malignant tumours of the adrenal glands or sympathetic nervous system. The tumour may be present and widespread at birth, and more than a third of affected children will show signs in the first year of life. The tumour spreads to liver, lungs and bones; such a spread has occurred in more than two-thirds of all cases by the time of diagnosis. Treatment is with radiation, surgery and chemotherapy. Abdominal tumours and those which have spread to the bones have a poor prognosis; infants respond to treatment better than older children.

NEUROFIBROMATOSIS (von Recklinghausen's disease)
Neurofibromatosis is an inherited condition in which multiple fibromas (small lumps of disorganised fibrous tissues) grow along the nerves. If these fibromas grow in a limited space,

such as the spinal canal, they compress the nerves to cause pain and disability and will need to be cut out, but the majority of fibromas can be safely left.

NON-ACCIDENTAL INJURY (BATTERING)
Non-accidental injury is the term given to injuries inflicted upon a child. Unexplained fractures, excessive bruising, sexual abuse and injuries to parts of the body seldom otherwise injured (e.g. recurrent black eyes, abdominal bruising, injuries inside the mouth) all arouse suspicion of non-accidental injury. This is only part of the broader spectrum of CHILD ABUSE.

OCCUPATIONAL THERAPY
Occupational therapists work with disabled children to help them to learn to do the activities of normal daily life, such as feeding, drawing and writing, dressing, and looking after themselves. Their patients may be children with developmental handicap, or children recovovering from accidents or surgery.

OPHTHALMOLOGIST
Ophthalmologists are medically qualified specialists in diseases and disorders of the eye. They work in hospitals and prescribe both medical and surgical treatment.

ORTHODONTIST
An orthodontist is a dentist concerned principally with the correction of misalignment and irregularities of the teeth. Correction of such irregularities improves the appearance, and can prevent the development of inaccessible areas of stagnation which may cause tooth decay. Orthodontists look after children with malocclusion (faulty alignment of the teeth which

causes an inefficient bite), secondary to prominent lower jaws, protruding upper incisors or crowding of the teeth. They are also involved in the care of children with cleft palates.

ORTHOPTIST
An orthoptist is a person qualified to detect and measure squints in children, to measure the visual acuity of each eye and to train the eye muscles. Orthoptists and ophthalmologists work together in hospitals. When the *ophthalmologist* (eye surgeon) prescribes orthoptic treatment for a squint, the orthoptist initiates a series of muscular exercises designed to coordinate the movements of the eyes, so that eventually the squint disappears and full binocular vision is restored. Some children will need a combination of surgical and orthoptic treatment.

OSTEOGENESIS IMPERFECTA (Brittle bone disease)
There are two main types of osteogenesis imperfecta. When it is severe, babies are born with multiple fractures and they continue to have fractures, become deformed and die soon after birth. In the less severe form, fractures occur after infancy, but the tendency to break bones easily disappears after puberty. Deafness is a late feature in some sufferers.

OSTEOMYELITIS
Osteomyelitis is a bacterial infection of the bone. It can affect children of any age. The commonest sites are near the ends of the long bones. The child with osteomyelitis experiences pain, fever, and a poor appetite. The skin and tissues over the bone become hot, red and excruciatingly tender. Treatment

is with intravenous antibiotics and, when necessary, surgical drainage of the pus from the bone. A prolonged course of oral antibiotics completes recovery.

PERITONITIS
Peritonitis is inflammation of the peritoneum, the lining membrane of the abdominal cavity. It usually occurs as a complication of bowel disease such as appendicitis, and represents a spread of the infection. Treatment depends on the underlying cause of the peritonitis.

PERTHÉ'S DISEASE
Perthé's disease is a condition in which the head of the femur gives way following a reduction in its blood supply. It occurs in children between the ages of four and ten. Initial symptoms are pain in the affected hip, and a limp. The femoral head is revascularized and regrows over a period of approximately two years. During this time some authorities recommend that the bone should be relieved of all weight-bearing in order that the femoral head is not squashed as it grows; the value of this prolonged treatment in younger children (who tend to have a better prognosis) is controversial.

PHENYLKETONURIA
Phenylketonuria is a rare genetic disorder of amino-acid metabolism. Unless placed on a special diet, a baby with phenylketonuria will become mentally handicapped. To prevent this, every baby has a Guthrie test at the end of the first week of life.This is when a heel prick blood sample is put onto a piece of absorbent paper and sent to the laboratory for analysis. It is a very sensitive screening test which enables early detection and

treatment of the condition. Affected individuals develop normally if they stick to the diet.

PHYSIOTHERAPIST
A physiotherapist is a person trained in the physical treatment and rehabilitation of children. Physical therapy including exercises and manipulation, is given to children with cerebral palsy, muscular dystrophy and other neuromuscular disorders. Arthritic children also benefit from regular exercises under the supervision of a physiotherapist. **Those with acute or chronic chest** infections also need physical treatment to help clear the secretions retained in the lungs.

PICA
Pica is the habit of eating dirt or other unsuitable substances. Some children will eat crayons, pencils, toys and even worms. Pica may be associated with poisoning if noxious materials (eg lead paints) are ingested. Pica is more common in mentally handi-capped and emotionally deprived children, than in otherwise normal children. Its presence should therefore always give rise to a more general consideration of the child's well-being. Many normal children do however go through a brief phase of earth-tasting.

POLIOMYELITIS
Poliomyelitis is a virus infection of the nerves in the spinal cord which results in paralysis. The illness starts with a headache, fever and general malaise and the paralysis develops after a few days. If the respiratory muscles are involved, assistance with breathing is necessary. Later, there is some apparent recovery as unaffected muscles partly take over the lost functions. The paralysed muscles waste away,

leaving a thin flaccid limb. The legs are affected more than the arms.

Poliomyelitis is a preventable disease. The vaccine is given within the first year either by injection or on a sugar lump . Unfortunately, a number of babies are not being vaccinated at present because of parental fears over reactions to vaccines, particularly for whooping cough. The polio vaccine is safe to take, and should be given. Travel to developing countries may result in the non-vaccinated child contracting poliomyelitis.

PSYCHIATRIST
A psychiatrist is a medically qualified specialist in mental illness. Child psychiatrists frequently work as part of a team including PSYCHOLOGISTS, nurse and psychiatric social workers. Such a team knows and helps not only the child, but the whole family.

PSYCHOLOGIST
A psychologist is trained to assess behavioural patterns, to measure intelligence quotients (IQ) and developmental quotients (DQ), and to recognize specific learning difficulties. Children most frequently meet educational psychologists at school when particular problems arise with basic subjects, with attention span, or with behaviour. Psychologists also work in child guidance clinics, and as part of the team in child psychiatry units.

RHESUS INCOMPATABILITY
Rhesus incompatability can occur when a rhesus negative mother has her second or subsequent rhesus (Rh) positive baby. In the USA and United Kingdom about eighty five per cent of women are rhesus positive and fifteen per cent are rhesus negative (see

BLOOD GROUPS). In any pregnancy in which a rhesus negative mother is carrying a rhesus positive baby, small amounts of positive blood may leak into her circulation, particularly during labour. This small innoculation of blood can sensitize the mother, who then develops antibodies against the rhesus positive factor. In subsequent pregnancies the antibodies will pass via the placenta into the baby's bloodstream and break down (haemolyse) his rhesus positive cells. This process is called rhesus haemolytic disease of the newborn. In mild cases there is only jaundice and slight anaemia after birth, but in more severe cases (now rarely seen) the baby will also be bloated with retained fluid (Hydrops foetalia) and suffer heart failure. Treatment of the more severe form is by exchange transfusion.

Although only about ten per cent of rhesus negative mothers develop antibodies, it is important to prevent this condition. For this reason all rhesus negative mothers are given an injection of Anti-D after the birth of their babies. 'D' is a principal part of the rhesus factor, and 'anti-D' is an antibody which 'mops up' any circulating baby cells before they can sensitize the mother. Thus the mother will not make her own antibodies and future pregnancies are protected.

RHEUMATIC FEVER
Rheumatic fever is now very rare in developed countries. It occurs after streptococcal infections. There may be a rapidly changing blotchy pink rash. The joints are affected and characteristically the pain and swelling moves from one joint to another. The heart may also be involved. Treatment consists of bed rest, aspirin to alleviate the symptoms, and penicillin to eradicate any persisting streptococcal infection. Recovery of the joints is complete, but the heart valves may be permanently damaged. Very rarely the central nervous system is involved and the resultant involuntary movements are known as St. Vitus's dance, or chorea.

RICKETS
Rickets is defective growth of the bones due to vitamin D deficiency. It results in the softening, bowing and widening of the long bones, ribs and skull. The widening of the bones may be apparent as swelling at the wrists, ankles and the ends of the ribs. The disease is rare nowadays because fortified milks and baby foods, containing adequate amounts of vitamin D, can be obtained.

Nevertheless rickets is occasionally seen in children whose diet is inadequate, and who have little exposure to sunlight which stimulates production of vitamin D.

ROSEOLA INFANTUM
Roseola infantum is an infectious disease of childhood in which a red rash develops over the body after two or three days of fever and malaise.

As soon as the rash appears the patient will start to improve.

SCABIES
Scabies is a skin infestation caused by a mite. It appears most commonly as an itchy rash on the wrists, hands, ankles and feet, but it can occur anywhere. A secondary infection, when the child has scratched the lesions leads to increased inflammation and weeping scabs. Treatment of scabies is in the form of an application of lotion all over the body for two successive nights with careful washing of all dirty clothes and bed linen. The itching subsides within a week of treatment.

SCARLET FEVER
Scarlet fever is a streptococcal infection. Sudden onset of fever, sore throat, general malaise with vomiting and the appearance of the characteristic rash typify an attack. The rash starts at the neck, armpits and groin and spreads rapidly. The face is flushed, the tongue at first white and furry, by the end of the week is bright red (strawberry tongue). Treatment is with penicillin. Aspirin or paracetamol can be given as necessary.

Scarlet fever is now uncommon as improved living conditions and hygiene, antibiotics and a natural reduction in the virulence of STREPTOCOCCI have all reduced its incidence and severity. When complications do occur, the heart, joints and kidneys may be involved.

SEPTICAEMIA
Septicaemia is a critical condition in which the life of the patient is threatened by a widespread infection of bacteria and their toxins circulating in the blood. The patient may need intensive care with antibiotics, intravenous fluids, and the maintenance of blood pressure and cardiac output, renal function and respiration.

SINUSITIS
The facial sinuses are not present at birth. The maxillary sinuses are hollows inside the bones of the face which develop at about the age of five. They connect up with the nose and may become infected. Persistent nasal catarrh may result. The frontal sinuses in

the bone of the forehead develop at about the age of twelve. They rarely become infected, but if they do, the condition can cause headaches.

SOCIAL WORKERS
The majority of social workers are based in the community, but a few are attached to specific institutions such as hospitals. The role of the social workers in the care of children is wide-ranging. At an early age, children with fostering or adoption are placed with families through social work agencies. The social worker may give indirect help to a child by supporting a family with psychiatric, financial or housing problems. More direct help may be offered by placing a toddler in a suitable nursery to relieve stress on a family, by helping families whose children are handicapped or have special needs, by giving guidance in families whose children are considered to be 'at risk' of child abuse, and by involvement with families where truancy and other behaviour problems may be emerging in their growing children.

SOLVENT ABUSE — See GLUE SNIFFING

SPINA BIFIDA
Spina bifida is a congenital defect in which there is maldevelopment of the vertebral column and spinal cord and the surrounding tissues. The severe forms -myelomeningocoele, in which the nerve fibres of the cord are exposed, and meningocoele in which only the bulging meninges protect the cord - are most frequently associated with handicap. *Hydrocephalus* (enlargement of the head) may be present. In severe cases, the nerves to the legs, bladder and anus may be irreversibly damaged

at birth. Exposure of the cord predisposes to the development of MENINGITIS.

Surgery on the newborn baby can be extremely difficult. At best it can only preserve the function already present, it never results in improvement. Surgeons and paediatricians now have experience of the outcome of surgery and the quality of life which the child will lead. In consulation with the parents they are therefore able to reach a conclusion as to the most appropriate treatment for a baby with spina bifida.

After the birth of one child with spina bifida, parents face a one in twenty risk of their future babies being affected. The condition can be diagnosed antenatally and the pregnancy terminated if the parents wish. Current research suggests that multivitamin supplementation of the mother's diet before, during and after conception reduces the risk of recurrence. Work to confirm this is still in progress.

STAPHYLOCOCCI
Staphylococci are the bacteria which cause the majority of boils, styes, abscesses and superficial skin infection. They also cause pneumonia. Staphylococci provoke the formation of pus. In many people they are constantly present in the nose and on the skin. However serious infections occur only when the more virulent strains overcome the host's resistance. Most staphylococci found in hospitals have become resistant to penicillin, but they are killed by other more powerful antibiotics.

STERNOMASTOID TUMOUR
The sternomastoid muscles run from the mastoid processes behind the ears to the top of the sternum (breast bone) and

clavicles. Damage to the muscle at birth may result in a small lump of fibrous scar tissue being palpable in the muscle some weeks later. This is not malignant, but merely the result of injury. It usually disappears after several months. Sometimes a slightly distorted neck results from damage to the muscle, but this is easily corrected with mild physiotherapy which is best given by the mother, after instruction.

STEROIDS
Steroids are a group of drugs whose structure and function closely resembles those of some of the hormones secreted by the adrenal glands. In cases of adrenal insufficiency they are used as replacement therapy to achieve a physiological effect. When used to treat other conditions, such as asthma, nephrotic syndrome or leukaemia, much larger doses are used and side-effects become apparent. These include increased appetite and weight gain, raised blood pressure and, if used for long periods in high doses, softening of the bones and reduced height. They must therefore be used only under close medical supervision.

STICKY EYE
A slight sticky discharge from one or both eyes developing 24 hours or so after birth is not uncommon. It is usually because of a combination of mild infection and poor drainage of the eye by the tear duct. Regular cleaning with cotton wool swabs soaked in water or saline is usually sufficient. If the discharge persists, antibiotic ointments can be used. If the condition recurs, a blockage of the tear duct may be present, but as this tends to clear spontaneously after a few months, it is best initially to

continue regular cleaning of the eye.

STREPTOCOCCI
Streptococci are a group of virulent bacteria causing infections ranging from tonsillitis, ear infections and sore throats to pneumonias, septicaemias and scarlet fever. The vast majority of infections are trivial, but a few are more serious, and some may develop complications involving the joints and kidneys. These conditions arise because of complex immunological reactions to the streptococcus. Streptococci are killed by penicillin and many other antibiotics.

STUTTERING
Three or four per cent of school age children stutter for a period. The reaction of their parents is crucial, as asking the stutterer to repeat phrases worsens the condition. Speech therapy may be needed for older persistent stutterers, but for the majority the support of their parents is sufficient. This includes helping with any stress the child is facing, and possibly establishing a regular play or story time with the child each day to show increased support and interest. This may also enable the child to talk out any problems worrying him.

TETANUS (Lockjaw)
Tetanus occurs when the toxins of the tetanus bacteria affect the central nervous system. The nerve cells are easily excited by slight stimuli, and massive muscular spasms occur. Breathing may be seriously affected, and the spasms may be very severe. With modern intensive care facilities, recovery is the rule, but in developing countries thousands of babies and young children still die each year from the disease.

Tetanus bacteria are found in the soil, and may spread to infect the body from any dirty cuts or wounds. It is preventable by vaccination; tetanus toxoid being part of the triple and booster vaccines given to children.

THYROID GLAND
The thyroid gland is placed astride the windpipe in the neck. It secretes the hormone thyroxin. Enlargement of the gland is called a GOITRE.

THYROID DEFICIENCY (HYPOTHYROIDISM)
Congenital hypothyroidism occurs in one in 3300 babies; untreated it can lead to *cretinism*. In the newborn baby it can cause prolonged jaundice, sleepiness, poor feeding and slow growth. Screening programmes for congenital hypothyroidism are now being introduced, and the blood for this test is taken at the end of the first week, at the same time as the Guthrie test for PHENYLKETONURIA. Early detection and treatment of congenital hypothyroidism prevents cretinism and the mental deficiency which occurs with it. Hypothyroidism may develop later in childhood for a variety of reasons.

Treatment of all forms of hypothyroidism is with thyroxin replacement. Measurement of hormone levels in the blood indicate when adequate therapy is being given.

THYROGLOSSAL CYST
During development of the foetus, the thyroid gland moves down from its original position at the base of the tongue to its final position low in the neck. As it does so it leaves behind a duct which normally disappears in time. Sometimes it develops a cystic swelling at the front of the neck at any point in the track of the thyroid's descent. This is a thyroglossal cyst; treatment is excision.

TISSUE TYPING
Tissue typing is a process similar to, but more sophisticated than, blood grouping. Just as blood has to be cross-matched to prove its compatibility prior to transfusion, so tissues which are to be transplanted have to be of the same or similar type as that of the recipient. Tissue typing has also revealed a genetic basis for predisposition to certain diseases such as arthritis.

TONGUE TIE
Tongue tie occurs when the frenum (the tag of tissue between the under surface of the tongue and the floor of the mouth) is short and extends to the very tip of the tongue. As growth occurs the tie becomes looser. Surgery is never warranted in the newborn and is seldom necessary later.

TOY LIBRARY
A toy library is a collection of toys which may be borrowed just as books are from an ordinary library. It provides an inexpensive and convenient way to provide appropriate and stimulating toys for the growing and developing child. The use of the toys by handicapped or deprived children is particularly encouraged.

TRAVEL SICKNESS
Travel sickness is common in young children over the age of two or three. The motion of travelling upsets the organs of balance in the ear, and the condition is made worse by the excitement of the journey.

The jolting in the back of most modern cars is worse than in the front. If there are appropriate safety harnesses, the child may travel better in the front seat. The car should not be too hot or stuffy, and the child should sit facing forwards with a good view of the passing scenery. Reading is not helpful, but if the child can be entertained, it helps to keep his mind off the sense of sickness.

If vomiting is imminent, the car can be stopped without undue fuss and the child should be allowed to recover in the fresh air before continuing the journey. Making a fuss will only add to the child's upset and make him think more of his nausea.

Severely affected children can benefit from a proprietary tablet taken half an hour before travelling. Drowsiness and dryness of the mouth are the usual side-effects of such medicines.

TURNER'S SYNDROME

Turner's syndrome occurs in 1 in 3,000 girls. The girl has only one X chromosome instead of the two required for normal female development. The ovaries are rudimentary and sexual maturation does not occur. Replacement hormone therapy in the early teens causes breast development but the girls are always infertile.

Features may be present at birth include oedema (puffiness) of the legs, webbing (loose floppy skin) of the neck, a low hairline and widely spaced nipples. Short stature is apparent later, and in some there may be mild mental retardation.

ULCERATIVE COLITIS

Ulcerative colitis is an inflammatory disease of the large bowel. Symptoms are abdominal pain, anorexia and nausea, and the passing of blood and mucousy stools. Treatment is with anti-inflammatory drugs, including steriods when

necessary. If active disease persists for a long period surgery may be indicated.

URTICARIA (nettle rash, hives)

Urticaria is a blotchy red swelling of the skin caused by the release of histamine in the affected areas. Histamine causes the small blood vessels to leak fluid into the tissue and this causes the characteristic rash. It is usually part of an allergic reaction, and if sensitivity to a particular food is apparent, it should be avoided. The rash can be soothed with calamine lotion, and topical or oral antihistamines may be beneficial.

VAGINAL DISCHARGE

A vaginal discharge of white mucus (the effect of maternal hormones), is normal in newborn girls and soon disappears. Older girls may have a smelly discharge if they have inserted something inside the vagina, or if they have an infecton. An inoffensive slight discharge is normal for a year or so prior to periods starting.

VERRUCAE

Verrucae are painful warts on the sole of the foot. The pressure on the foot tends to make the wart grow inwards and become tender. Verrucae spread in warm, moist conditions such as swimming pools and school showers. Soaking the affected area nightly in formalin and then rubbing down with sand-paper is one treatment; another is an application of podophyllin under a plaster. It may take weeks for the verrucae to disappear.

VITAMINS

Vitamins are organic nutrients present in only small quantities in a normal diet, but they are essential to life, growth and normal health. A mixed and varied diet provides adequate

amounts of all vitamins, but certain exclusion diets are deficient and need vitamin supplementation. Commercial infant milks are fortified with vitamins, but it is presently recommended that the exclusively breast-fed infant receives vitamin D supplements. See vitamin chart, page 31.

WARTS

Warts are caused by virus infections of the skin. The majority of warts resolve spontaneously if left alone and therefore no treatment is necessary. This is a hard course to follow as new warts tend to appear and may take several years to disappear. Warts most commonly appear on the hands and soles of the feet (see VERRUCAE). On the hands they can be treated by a dermatologist with a carbon dioxide 'snow stick', or by application of ointments, available over the counter or on prescription.

WILM'S TUMOUR (NEPHROBLASTOMA)

Wilm's tumour is a rare malignant tumour of the kidney. It usually shows up in the first three years of life with a swollen abdomen and a palpable mass. Often fever, pain or blood in the urine are the first symptoms. Treatment is a combination of drug therapy, radiation and surgery. Prognosis is best with small unilateral tumours in young children. If there is no evidence of recurrence after two years, long term survival is probable.

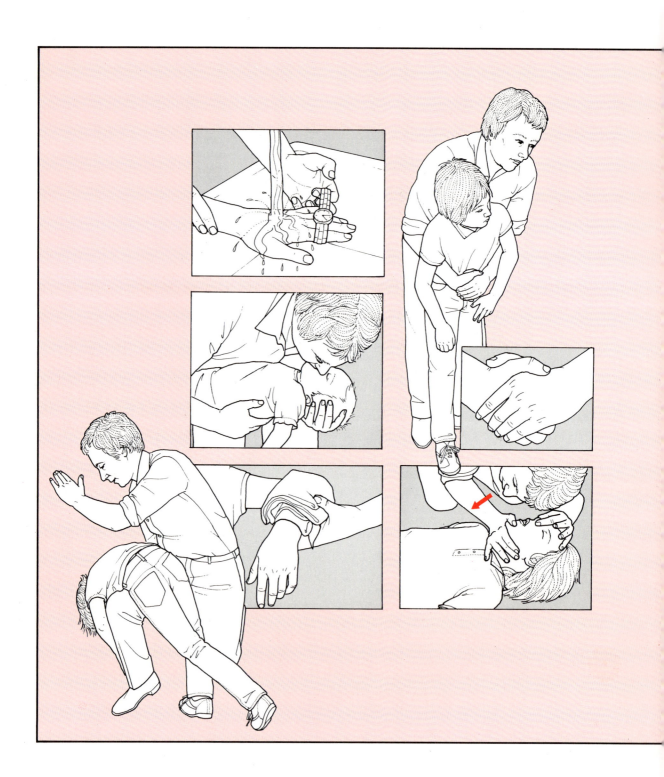

Section Four:
First Aid and Accident Prevention

All parents should know what to do in a
life-threatening situation. For example,
if a child has stopped breathing, is
suffering from severe bleeding or
is choking, some knowledge of the major
first aid techniques will enable the parent
to act immediately. This is very valuable in a
situation where every minute counts. If
medical help is going to be required
first aid treatment should be confined to
the minimum necessary to make the patient
comfortable and to protect the injured part.
Also contained in this section is
an A-Z of first aid steps for treating
minor injuries, information about accident
prevention and safety in the home,
and a list of what to keep in a first aid box.

Safety and Accident Prevention

CHILDREN ARE GREAT EXPLORERS and adventurers and need to be protected, as far as is reasonably possible, from serious falls, scalds and burns, swallowing tablets which look like sweets, and chemical substances which look like drinks. They need to learn road safety drills and to be aware of the environmental dangers which face them when away from home. Above all they need parental supervision until they are old enough to care for themselves. Surveys have reported that some parents consider children aged two or three years, old enough to cross busy roads. This is clearly inappropriate, for many children do not have an adequate sense of safety on the roads or in other places until they are ten years old or more.

Prevention, as always, is better than cure. Homes in which there are young children need special features to reduce the risk of accidents. Stairs should be well lit, with safety gates at both the top and bottom for very young children. There should not be gaps between the railings on the landings as infants can wriggle through these and fall into the well of the stairs. Windows, particularly those in high rise flats, need safety catches to prevent opening to the point which would allow a child to fall out. Windows reaching to the floor, patio doors and glass in the lower panels of doors should all be made of safety glass. This glass is highly resistant to impact and therefore less likely to break and cut a child who is falling. Children can be badly scalded by hot drinks. This can cause scarring injuries to the face and other parts of the body and is easily avoided by keeping hot substances out of the reach of the child. Electrical burns are severe and all appliances and their flexes should be checked regularly to prevent both burns and shocks.

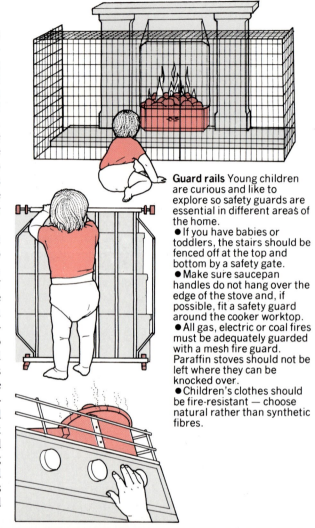

Guard rails Young children are curious and like to explore so safety guards are essential in different areas of the home.
- If you have babies or toddlers, the stairs should be fenced off at the top and bottom by a safety gate.
- Make sure saucepan handles do not hang over the edge of the stove and, if possible, fit a safety guard around the cooker worktop.
- All gas, electric or coal fires must be adequately guarded with a mesh fire guard. Paraffin stoves should not be left where they can be knocked over.
- Children's clothes should be fire-resistant — choose natural rather than synthetic fibres.

Road safety Children are vulnerable as pedestrians, as cyclists and as passengers. Note the following:-
- Never allow young children out into the road unaccompanied. Keep toddlers on walking reins when you are out and start to teach your children road sense as soon as they are able to understand instructions.
- If your child has a bicycle, make sure it is properly maintained. Don't allow children to ride on the road until they are competent and never let a child ride a bike that is too big (see right) for him to cope with.
- When you take children out in the car, make sure that they are secured safely in the back seat (see page 171).

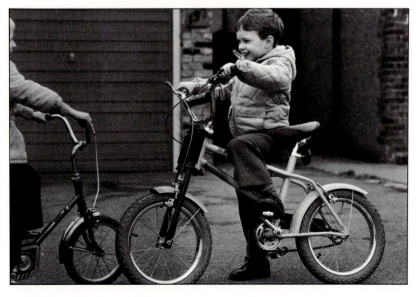

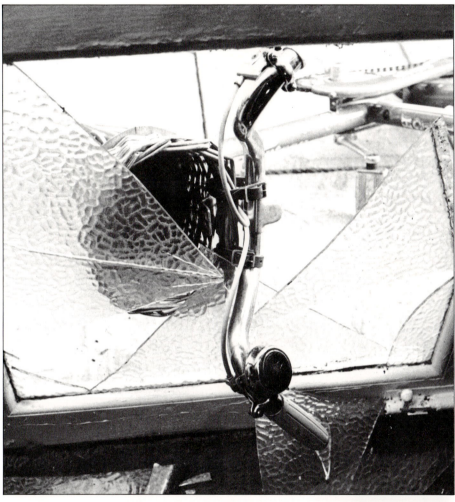

Windows and glazing

Accidents with glass are not uncommon and can cause the most serious cuts. Children can be hurt badly from a fall through or into a glass door or window, so the following precautions should be taken:-
● Do not place furniture where children can easily climb up to an open window.
● Wherever possible, fit safety glass in your home. It is highly resistant to impact and is less likely to cause injury.

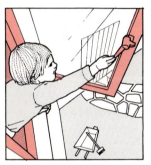

Safety locks/bars Special locks and catches on doors and windows can be fitted easily. If a window is particularly dangerous window bars can be put on, but make sure they can be removed in case of fire.
● Fit safety catches to upstairs windows so that the child cannot open the window.
● Do not allow children onto a balcony unattended.

As the child gets older try to teach him what situations are dangerous and help him to use his judgement so that he avoids taking unnecessary risks.

If the child likes adventure sports, such as rock climbing, sailing or pony treking, make sure he is taught properly, has the right equipment and practises the sport in a safe place.

Children who have roller skates or skate boards are better off going to a park or rink, rather than skating in the road or on the pavement. Most areas have facilities for skaters and the child should be encouraged to make use of them.

Water

Children love to play in or near water, but there is always a danger of drowning so watch them very carefully.
● At the seaside or in a swimming pool keep an eye on children, particularly if they cannot swim. If they are

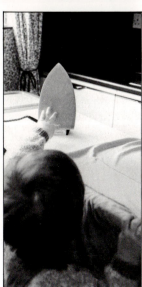

Electrical appliances Small children are at particular risk from burns and scalds as they will touch anything they can reach and do not understand about heat and fire.
● Irons, kettles and other electrical appliances get very hot. Do not leave them where children can touch them.
● Cover electric sockets with a safety cover or a dummy plug. Children are inclined to stick objects into the socket and could get a nasty shock.

still learning to swim they should wear arm bands or rubber rings to keep them afloat. Make sure they do not drift out beyond their depth.
● For sailing and canoeing, and other activities on the water, children should wear life jackets.
● Water tanks and barrels, and garden ponds, should be covered with wire mesh if there are young children about.
● Babies and toddlers must never be left alone in a bath — not even for a minute.

Preventing fires
Most house fires can be avoided and to reduce the risk of fire in the home note the following precautions:
● Always unplug the television, radio and stereo before going to bed.

● Empty ashtrays at the end of the day.
● Do not use a portable electric fire in the bathroom.
● Never leave matches lying around within a child's reach.
● Remember the risk of fire when cooking. Never leave a pan of hot oil or fat on the cooker unattended.

Action at a fire
If the house is on fire, get everybody out *immediately*. Fumes from burning materials can cause rapid asphyxiation. If it is a small fire, try to smother the flames with a rug or blanket.
If a pan of hot fat or oil catches fire, do not pour water over it. Turn the heat off and put a damp cloth or a lid over it to stop it from spreading. Then leave it to cool down.

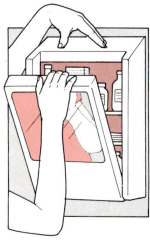

Medical cabinets Medicines should be kept out of reach of children, in a locked cabinet. Remember this when visiting or being visited by friends or relatives who may be on regular medication. Dispose of old, unwanted medicines down the toilet, NEVER in the dustbin.

Child-proof containers Medication can be kept in child-proof containers. The most common of these is the bottle with the top that has to be pushed down as it is turned. Children find these difficult, but by no means impossible to open and although useful they are no substitute for a locked cabinet.

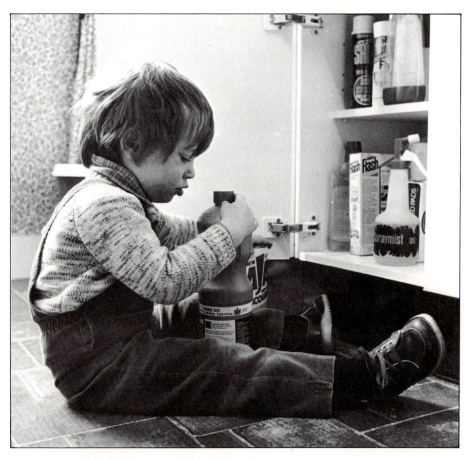

Poisonous substances Bleaches, disinfectants, paints, turpentine, weed killer and other chemicals should always be kept out of reach and locked up. NEVER use milk, or other soft drink bottles to store garden or household chemicals. Alcoholic drink can also be dangerous to young children. A lockable drinks cabinet is the safest place for intoxicating liquor. Never assume that something which smells or tastes horrible will not be consumed by a child; children will try anything and one gulp of a poisonous substance could cause permanent damage.

Safety in the car

It is very important for children to be adequately protected when travelling in a car and the use of proper car seats for children is absolutely essential for safety. Make sure and note the following precautions:-

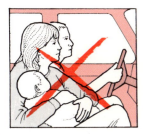

● Never put the child in the front passenger seat in the arms of a passenger. If the car stops suddenly, both adult and child will smash into or through the windscreen.
● Small children should not be placed in adult seatbelts — they could slip and catch the belt under the chin, causing throat or spinal injuries.
● Never let a child stand on the seat or lean out of the car window.
● Never put a child in the front seat of a car, **without a seatbelt**. If there is an accident, the child is liable to hit the windscreen or be thrown through it and could sustain severe head injuries, including scarring. The safest way for children to travel is properly secured in the back seat.

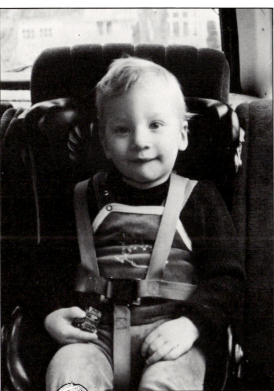

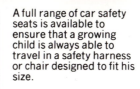

A full range of car safety seats is available to ensure that a growing child is always able to travel in a safety harness or chair designed to fit his size.

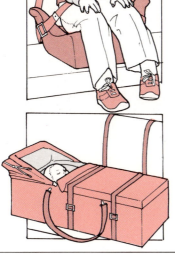

Babies can travel safely on the back seat of a car in a carry-cot which is strapped down to proper anchorage points.

Child locks can be fitted on the car doors to stop children from falling or climbing out.

Accident prevention checklist

Accidents are the most common cause of death for children over the age of one year and also a major cause of permanent handicap. Children must be protected from accidents and taught at an early age to recognize and cope with the dangers around them.
  Babies and toddlers are at particular risk so observe the following rules:
1. Never leave polythene bags laying around; a child might put it over his head and could suffocate.
2. Don't leave a baby alone feeding from a bottle.
3 Keep all medicines out of reach of children.
4. Don't let babies play with very small objects, such as beads or buttons — they can choke very easily.
5. Straps, strings or ribbons around a child's neck can pull and cause strangulation.
6. Teach children not to pick and eat plants or seeds — they could be poisonous.
7. Broken glass often causes nasty cuts, so be sure to clear broken glass away promptly, particularly if you have a toddler or baby who is crawling.
8. Do not let small children walk or run with bottles or glasses they may fall over and cut themselves.
9. Keep sharp tools away from toddlers.
10. Never leave a child unattended in a bath or near a garden pond which is not fenced off.
11. Keep toys out of the kitchen — you could trip and fall while carrying something hot or heavy.

A Matter of Life and Death
Emergency techniques

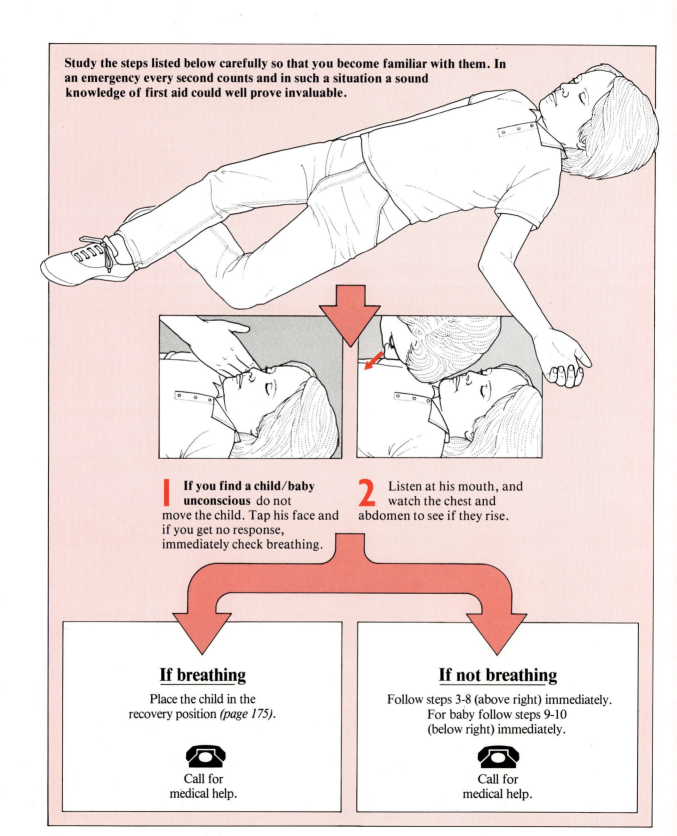

Study the steps listed below carefully so that you become familiar with them. In an emergency every second counts and in such a situation a sound knowledge of first aid could well prove invaluable.

1 **If you find a child/baby unconscious** do not move the child. Tap his face and if you get no response, immediately check breathing.

2 Listen at his mouth, and watch the chest and abdomen to see if they rise.

If breathing

Place the child in the recovery position *(page 175)*.

Call for medical help.

If not breathing

Follow steps 3-8 (above right) immediately. For baby follow steps 9-10 (below right) immediately.

Call for medical help.

Mouth-to-mouth respiration CHILD

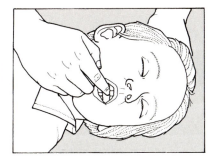

3 Place the child on his back. Turn the head to one side and clear the mouth of any vomit, blood, loose teeth or other objects. If breathing starts, place in the recovery position *(page 175)*.

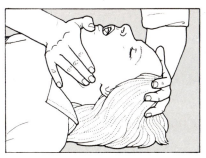

4 If still not breathing, arch the neck and tilt the head back, holding the forehead and chin. Open the mouth. (If the mouth is damaged, do mouth-to-nose respiration. Close off the mouth and breath into his nose).

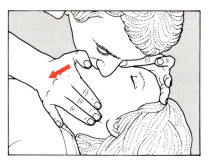

5 Take a deep breath and place your open mouth over the child's mouth. Pinch the nostrils closed with your fingers and give five good breaths into his mouth. Watch to see if the chest rises as you do this.

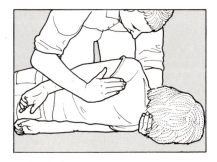

6 If the chest does not rise check the mouth again for blockage. Pull the child towards you, onto his side, and slap him twice between the shoulder blades.

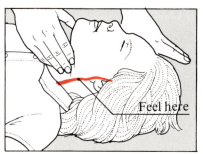

7 Check the pulse on the child's neck. If a pulse is felt, give two good breaths into his mouth. (If there is no pulse consider heart massage, *page 174*, in conjunction with mouth-to-mouth respiration).

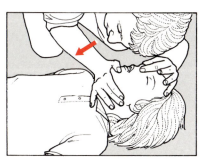

8 Continue breathing into his mouth every five seconds until breathing starts or medical aid is obtained. If breathing does restart place in the recovery position *(page 175)*.

Mouth-to-mouth respiration BABY

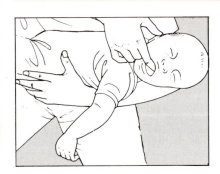

9 Lay the baby on his back and tilt the head back. Support the head and turn it to one side. Check that the baby's mouth is clear. If necessary, carefully clear the baby's mouth of any vomit or objects with a finger.

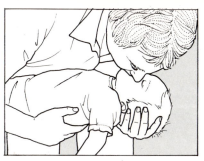

10 Cover the baby's mouth and nose with your own mouth and blow gently into the lungs at twenty breaths per minute. After the first four breaths check to see if the chest and abdomen are rising. If there is no sign of breathing continue mouth-to-mouth respiration until breathing starts, or medical aid is obtained. If no heart beat is apparent, consider heart massage *(page 174)*.

If you find an unconscious child always check for medical clues. Children who suffer from a particular condition (for example diabetes) will probably wear a 'medic alert' braciet.

Heart Massage CHILD

Do not start heart massage unless you are sure the heart has stopped. It can cause damage.

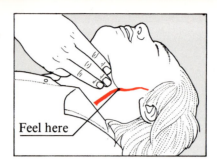

1 Check to see if you can feel a pulse in the neck. If you can, heart massage is not needed.

Feel here

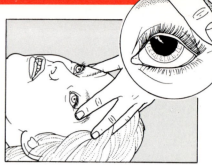

2 Check eyes; if the heart has stopped the pupils will be dilated.

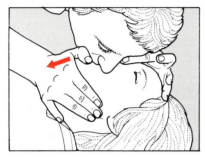

3 If the heart is not beating, place the child on his back on a firm surface and give him two good breaths of mouth-to-mouth respiration. Check again to see if the heart is beating. If you are sure it is not, start heart massage in conjunction with mouth-to-mouth respiration.

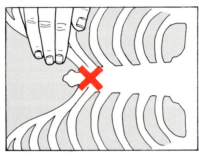

4 Stand or kneel beside the child's chest. Locate the massage point by running your hand up the inside of the rib cage until you feel the breastbone. The massage point is just above this, as indicated in the diagram by a cross. Place the heel of one hand on the massage point.

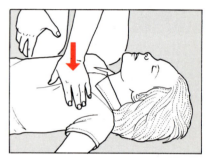

5 With your arm straight, press down firmly so that the breast bone moves about an inch (2.5cm), and then relax. Repeat about once a second. After 15 presses give two breaths of mouth-to-mouth respiration, then restart heart massage until recovery, or medical aid arrives.

Heart Massage BABY

Do not start heart massage unless you a sure the heart has stopped. It can cause damage.

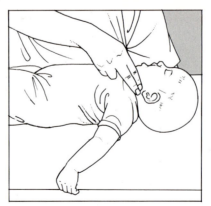

1 Place the baby on his back on a firm surface and check to see if you can feel a pulse in the neck. If you can, heart massage is not needed.

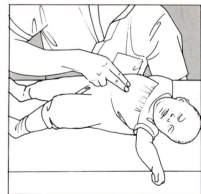

2 If the heart is not beating use two fingers to apply firm pressure to the breastbone, approximately 80 times a minute.

The recovery position

This is the correct position for an unconscious child who is still breathing.
It is comfortable, makes breathing easier and prevents the tongue from falling to the back of the throat and obstructing the airway. This sequence illustrates turning a child who is lying on his back — you will have to adapt the procedure if the body is in a different position.

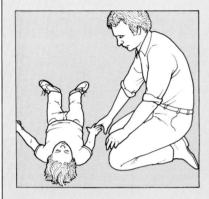

1 Kneel beside the child at chest level. Loosen restrictive clothing and, if the child is wearing spectacles, take them off.

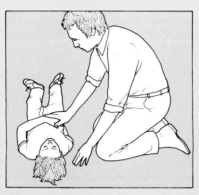

2 Place the child's arms nearest to you, under the buttocks, with the palm upwards. Bring the other arm across the chest.

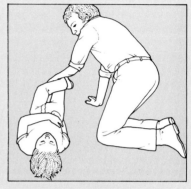

3 Cross the child's leg, farthest from you, over the other leg.

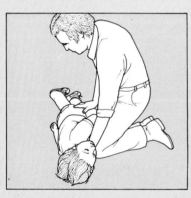

4 Taking care to protect the child's head, roll him towards you and support him against your knees.

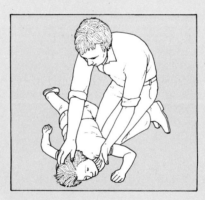

5 Bend the child's uppermost leg at the knee to support the lower part of the body. Place the uppermost arm beside the head. Gently pull the other arm out to lie parallel to the body.

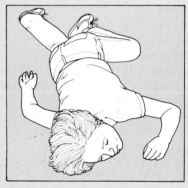

6 Carefully lift the head up and back to aid breathing.

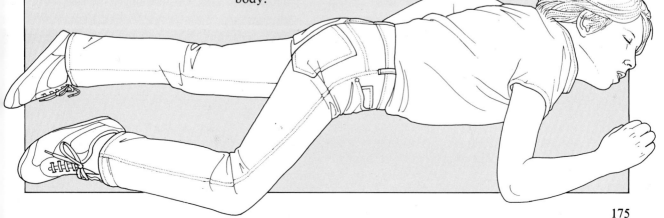

A-Z of First Aid

First aid steps for treating injuries and illness are described and illustrated on the following pages. These instructions can be used as a guideline for treating the child, preventing the condition from worsening, providing effective relief and making the child as comfortable as possible until placing him, if necessary, in the care of a doctor or taking him to a hospital. For some minor injuries, such as blisters and abrasions, first aid may be all that is needed.

The more knowledge a person has of first aid the better and the information given in this section should not be seen as a substitute for practical first-aid training. However, provided you are able to assess the situation correctly, and follow the appropriate steps accurately and quickly, then the information given here will prove very useful.

Abrasions/Grazes

These usually result from a sliding fall which scrapes the top layer of skin, leaving a raw area underneath. This type of wound often contains dirt or grit and, although it is minor, it can become infected. The aim, therefore, is to clean and dress the wound as soon as possible. Lightly wash the graze and cover it with a sterile dressing of a suitable size.

Bleeding

Bleeding may occur externally or internally. If the blood loss is heavy, the face and lips become pale, the skin is cold and clammy, the pulse gets weak. This is known as shock. *(page 182)*. Fainting may also occur as a result of blood loss *(page 179)*. If blood loss has been significant, seek medical aid or transfer the child to hospital.

If breathing has stopped, start mouth-to-mouth ventilation *(page 173)* as well as attending to bleeding.

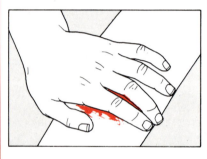

Severe external bleeding
1. Apply prolonged pressure over the wound after first removing any obvious foreign bodies.

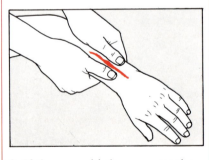

2. If the wound is large, press the edges together gently and maintain pressure.

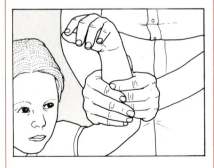

3. If possible, lower the child's head and raise the bleeding part.

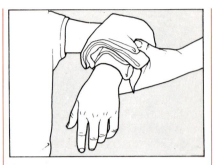

4. Prepare a sterile dressing which will more than cover the wound. Cover with a soft pad and bandage around firmly.

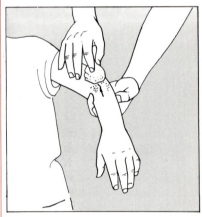

Minor external bleeding
1. Apply an antiseptic lotion to the wound repeatedly until any visible dirt particles have been washed away.
2. Apply a large firm dressing to the wound.
3. Ensure that a tetanus toxoid booster is given after all deep or dirty wounds if the injured child has not had one for *two years* or more. Deep wounds may only bleed a little, but are prone to infection, and tetanus precautions are particularly important.

Internal bleeding
Look out for signs of faintness, rapid pulse rate, cold sweaty skin, thirst, or rapid breathing after an accident. These could be signs of internal bleeding. Medical advice must be sought.

Blisters

Blisters caused by friction, such as rubbing from new shoes, need to be kept clean, and covered with a protective dressing.
1. **Do not** burst the blister if it has not already broken.
2. Cover with a clean dressing.
3. Put on some padding, and hold in place with a plaster or bandage.

Burns and scalds

The severity of a burn depends both on the area and the depth. Loss of plasma and fluids from a large burn can send a child into shock. *See treatment of shock, page 182*.

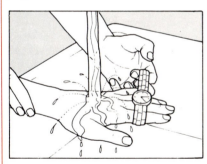

1. Immediately immerse the burnt part in cold running water for several minutes. This cools the tissues and limits the extent of the injury.
2. Remove watches, jewellery and tight clothes from around the burnt area to prevent swelling.
3. Apply a clean dressing and secure with a loose bandage. **Do not** break blisters or touch the injury.
4. Seek medical advice for all but the smallest burns.

Chemical burns
Wash in cold water until the chemical is completely flushed away. Remove contaminated clothing whilst continuing to wash

burns. Seek medical aid.

Acid and caustic burns to the eye *See eye injuries, page 179*.

Clothes on fire
Lay the child down to stop the flames sweeping upwards to the face. Quickly throw water over the flames. Alternatively wrap the child tightly in a blanket or heavy fabric and lay on the ground. **Do not** roll the child as this can cause spreading of the burns.

Electrical burns
Turn off the appliance and observe the precautions detailed under electric shock *(page 179)*. Attend to the burns only when satisfied that the breathing and circulation are satisfactory. *See resuscitation techniques, page 173*.

Mouth and throat burns
Transfer a child who has inhaled smoke or flames to hospital.

Choking

Choking normally occurs when the airway is partially or totally blocked. It is essential that any obstruction is removed quickly.

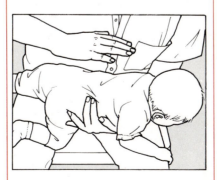

Babies
1. Hold the baby with his head down, supporting his chest and abdomen. Slap the baby smartly between the shoulder blades up to four times, but not too hard.

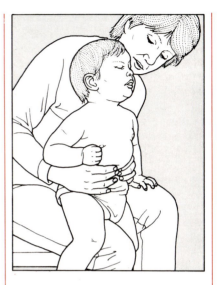

2. If this does not dislodge the object, sit the baby on your lap. Put the tips of two fingers of each hand side-by-side slightly above the baby's navel. Press gently but firmly upwards.

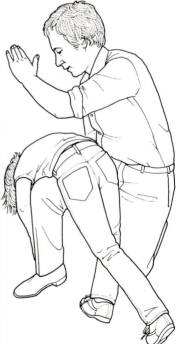

Children
1. Quickly remove any blood, vomit, teeth or other objects from the child's mouth. Lay the child over your knee with the head

down. With one hand support the chest and with the other slap the child briskly between the shoulder blades, up to four times. If this does not dislodge the obstruction, proceed to step 2.

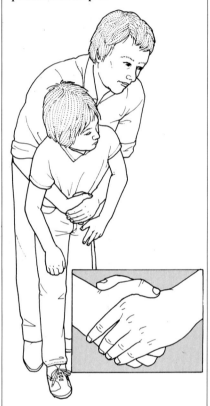

2. Stand behind the child and wrap both arms around the stomach. Grasp the hands together and suddenly and sharply squeeze the stomach.

If the child is unconscious place on a firm surface and roll him onto one side. Slap him twice between the shoulder blades. Check to see if the obstruction has been dislodged. If it has not, turn the child over and start mouth-to-mouth ventilation *(page 173)*.

Convulsions/Fits

Fits can occur because of epilepsy, infection, fever or poisoning. If a child is having a fit, follow this procedure.

1. Place in the recovery position *(page 175)*.
2. **Do not** attempt to force the mouth open if it is tightly closed.
3. Wipe away saliva and vomit.
4. Summon medical help or take the child to hospital.
5. Take measures to cool the child if he is feverish.

Cramp

Cramp is a sudden and painful contraction of a muscle or muscles. It can occur during exercise such as swimming, or be due to loss of salt or water from the body.

1. Feet and hands: straighten out the child's toes or fingers and massage gently.
2. Thigh or calf: straighten the knee, gently raise the leg and push the child's foot up towards the shin. Gently massage the affected muscles. *(See below)*

Dog bites

1. Wash the wound with water and a mild antiseptic solution until it is clean.
2. Look carefully for penetrating wounds which may be difficult to clean.
3. Apply a clean unmedicated dressing.
4. Take the child to the doctor or nearest hospital for assessment of the wound and for a tetanus booster (if none has been given in the last two years).
In some parts of the world a course of vaccinations against rabies has to be considered. Seek medical advice.

Drowning

If a large volume of any kind of water is inhaled, major breathing difficulties will ensue.

Resuscitation of a drowned person needs to be started as soon as possible.

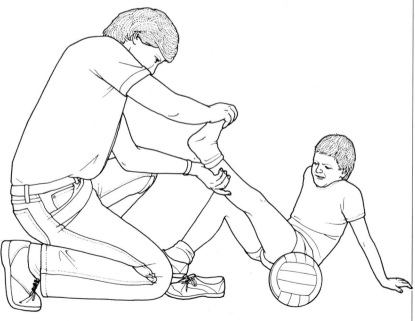

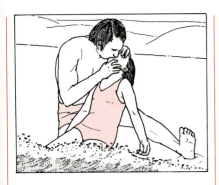

In the water
With a small child, mouth-to-mouth breathing *(page 173)* can be done whilst still in the water, and full resuscitation should be started as soon as you are back on firm ground.
On land
Start full resuscitation immediately. All victims of near-drowning need immediate hospitalization. Lung infections and chemical disturbances in the body are later complications which can be life threatening.

Electric shock

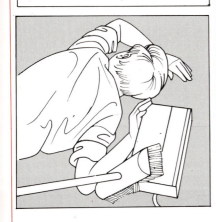

Domestic
1. Do not touch the child until you have switched off the electricity and pulled him clear.
   If the electricity cannot be turned off, use a broom handle to push the child clear of the contact. Make sure you are not standing on a wet surface.

2. Check heartbeat and breathing. Start resuscitation if necessary *(see page 173)*.
3. Once breathing is satisfactory, attend to any burns *(see page 177)*.

NB If the child is in contact with a high voltage source, such as a railway line or pylon, **do not** attempt a rescue until the power supply has been switched off. High voltages can jump distances.

Eye injuries

If there has been any penetration of the eyeball (eg flying glass), take the child to hospital immediately.

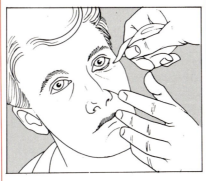

Minor foreign bodies on the conjunctiva
1. Put the child under a good light and lift off the particle with the moistened tip of a clean handkerchief or tissue.

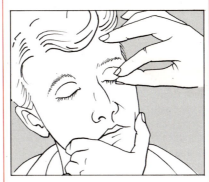

2. If it is stuck to the undersurface of the upper lid, gently hold the lid

and, with the child looking down, rub it gently over the lower lid.
3. If this does not dislodge the particle, a matchstick may be placed in the fold of the upper lid and the eyelid pulled over it if the child is cooperative. The particle can then be removed with the moistened tip of a handkerchief. The lid will return to its normal position when released.
4. If you cannot remove an obstruction from the eye, cover the eye with an eye pad, secure it in position and seek medical aid.

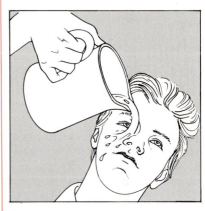

Acid and caustic burns of the eyes
Hold the child's head under cold water for several seconds. Make sure the child blinks and opens the eye while you are doing this. Transfer the child to hospital immediately, while continuing to wash the eye.

Black eye
Reduce swelling and pain with a cold damp cloth. Consult a doctor if you think there has been any serious damage to the eye or surrounding bone.

Fainting

Fainting results from a temporary insufficiency of the blood supply to the brain. Fright, pain or shock can cause fainting. Recovery occurs within minutes.

If a child is going to faint or when he has come round:

1. Encourage deep breathing.

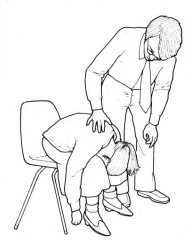

2. Sit the child down and place the head between the knees, or lie him down with the feet up.
3. Loosen clothing.
4. Make sure that the child has plenty of fresh air.
5. When completely recovered, give small sips of cold water.

Foreign bodies

Ears/nose

If a foreign body, such as a bead or peanut, becomes lodged in the ear or nose, take the child to hospital for the removal to be done by an expert. Attempted removal without the correct instrument often pushes the object further in and can cause damage. Insects: If an insect becomes lodged in the ear, it can be washed out by flooding the ear with warm water.

Throat

If a fishbone, or other object, feels as though it is stuck in the throat seek medical advice. *See choking, page 177.*

Eyes

See eye injuries, page 178.

Fractures and dislocations

Fractures can occur as the result of a fall or with other injuries in a traffic accident. When there are other injuries, deal with breathing, bleeding and major problems first.

The signs of a fracture are pain or tenderness, swelling and sometimes deformity. There is also loss of normal movement. If a fracture is suspected, medical aid should be sought. Therefore perform the minimum of first aid necessary, and do not give the child anything to eat or drink in case the bones have to be set under a general anaesthetic.

A dislocation occurs when a bone at the joint is wrenched into an abornormal position by a sudden movement or fall. Joints which are most commonly dislocated are the elbow, the thumb, the knee and the jaw. The injured joint will usually look deformed and there will be swelling and bruising later on.

Dislocations should be treated by a doctor as the displaced joint must by put back into position. If there is no medical help available immediately try to make the child as comfortable as possible until professional help arrives.

It is often difficult to distinguish between a disclocation and a fracture, so if you are in any doubt and have to move the child, treat as a fracture.

The arm

If the suspected fracture is in the arm, place it in a sling and take the child to hospital. Described below are steps on how to apply an arm sling. This sling holds the forearm across the chest but it is only effective if the child sits or stands.

With all suspected fractures in

the arm check that you can feel the wrist pulse. If not, gently move the arm into the extended position and feel the pulse again. If it is now present, leave the arm in this position. Do not move the arm if the child resists or it appears to be causing extreme pain.

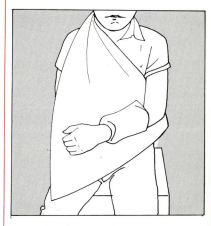

To make an arm sling
1. Ask the child to sit down. Support the arm by the wrist and hand or get the child to support his own arm. Wrap padding around the injured arm.

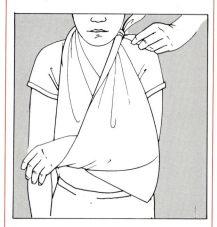

2. Continue to support the arm by the wrist and slide one end of the triangular bandage between the chest and forearm so that its point reaches well below the elbow. Bring the top end over the shoulder on the sound side and around the back of the neck.

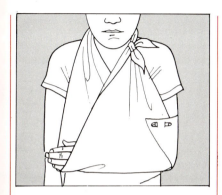

3. Continue to support the arm and bring the lower end of the bandage over the hand and forearm. Tie with a knot above the collar bone. Secure the point of the sling around the elbow with a safety pin.

The leg
A fracture in the leg can be in the upper limb (the thigh bone or femur) or the lower limb (the tibia or fibula). If you have to move the child yourself, immobilize and support the injured leg with a splint. Try to move the injured part as little and as carefully as possible when treating the fracture.

To make a splint
If there is no plank of wood available you can use fencing, sticks, a broom handle, rolled up newspaper or any suitable padding to make an improvised splint.

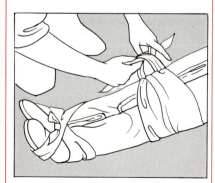

1. For a fracture in the lower leg, place the splint between the legs

from ankle to crotch. If possible, put padding around it to make it more comfortable for the child. Tie a figure of eight bandage around the feet and ankles to secure the splint.

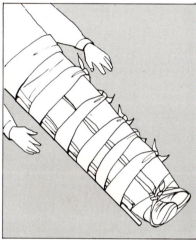

2. For a fracture in the upper limb, place one splint between the legs with padding and another along the outside of the injured leg, from ankle to armpit. Tie a figure of eight bandage around the feet and ankles. Tie three or four other bandages around the shin, knee and thigh and tie them on the uninjured side.

Fractures in special places
Spine: 1. Do not move the child unless there is immediate threat to life. *See traffic accidents, page 183.*
2. Call the ambulance service immediately.
3. If the child is conscious, try to find out if he is able to move his fingers and toes, and whether sensation in them seems normal. Prevent him from moving any other parts of his body.
4. Give nothing my mouth.

Elbow: Fractures involving the elbow are common in children. If the elbow cannot be bent:

1. Lay the child down and place the injured arm by his body. Do not attempt to bend the elbow.
2. Place soft padding between the injured arm and the body.

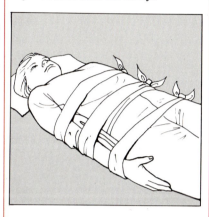

3. Secure the arm to the body by three broad bandages, around the wrist and thighs, around the upper arm and body, around the forearm and body.
4. Take the child to hospital, maintaining the treatment position.

Face and jaw: 1. Keep the airway clear.
2. Gently remove blood, vomit and loose teeth from the mouth.

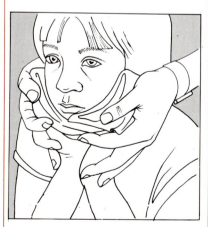

3. Support the jaw gently with one hand, or with a pad or bandage secured at the top of the head.
4. Transfer to hospital as soon as possible.

Head injuries

Injuries to the scalp tend to cause profuse bleeding. If the scalp is cut or split, the bleeding can be controlled with pressure. If the skin is not broken, bleeding under the scalp may form a large bruise. Eventually the pressure of the bruise helps to stop the bleeding and no action is necessary.

Loss of consciousness
If the child has only a brief period when he is pale and quiet following a head injury, there is no need to worry, but if the child is unconscious:
1. Place in the recovery position.
2. Check heartbeat and breathing, and resuscitate if necessary *(page 173)*.
3. Seek medical aid.
   If a child has had a head injury, whether or not there has been unconsciousness, the following should cause concern:
● Slurred speech or abnormal movements.
● A convulsion.
● Persistent vomiting.

If any of these occur, the child should be taken to hospital. Be prepared for the child to be admitted for investigation or observation.

Insect stings

1. Remove the sting, if present, with a pair of tweezers.
2. Apply an antihistamine cream or calamine lotion.
3. If the sting is in the mouth, sucking ice may help.
4. If swelling in the mouth occurs which begins to affect breathing, give ice to suck and transfer to a casualty department.
5. For jellyfish stings, soothe with a little calamine lotion.

Nose bleeds

These can be caused by accidents involving a blow to the face, but spontaneous nosebleeds are common in all children.

1. Pinch the nostrils for 5 to 10 minutes.
2. Allow the child to breath through an open mouth.
3. Keep the child's head forward. If the child swallows blood it can cause vomiting.
4. Seek medical advice if the bleeding persists.

Poisoning

Try and find out quickly what substance has been taken.
Do not induce vomiting if the child has taken petroleum products, kerosene, turpentine, bleach, caustic or acid compounds. If any of the above have been taken, give the child milk to drink and take him to a casualty department immediately or summon an ambulance.

In suspected poisoning with other substances, if the child is conscious try and induce vomiting.
To make a child vomit give a large drink and then stick one or two fingers down the throat. Do not waste time if this proves difficult, but transfer the child to a hospital casualty department.
If the child is unconscious do not induce vomiting. Place in the recovery position with the head down to stop vomit being inhaled. Transfer urgently to a casualty department.

Late discovery of poisoning Even if the poisonous substance was taken some hours previously, act promptly, and as above.

Shock

Shock following an injury can be very serious and is caused by loss of blood or other fluids from the body, abdominal injury or fright.
1. Comfort and reassure the child.
2. Loosen tight clothing and cover the child with a blanket or coat.
3. Do not give anything to drink, but moisten the lips with water if the child is thirsty.
4. If breathing is difficult, place in the recovery position. If breathing has stopped, begin mouth-to-mouth breathing *(page 173)*.
4. Remove to hospital.

Snake bites

Bites from venomous snakes are of varying severity, depending on the snake, the amount of venom injected and the victim's state of health. Snake bites in children are serious, and medical aid should be obtained immediately.
1. Immobilize the bitten part to slow down absorption of the venom.
2. Cover the wound with a dry dressing.
3. Transport to hospital quickly, preferably in a lying position.

Do not apply a tourniquet, suck out or incise the wound, or apply any chemicals to the bite.

Sprains

When a joint is forcibly stretched beyond its limits there may be damage to tissues around the joint. Sprains may arise from falling awkwardly, or tripping whilst running.
   The affected joint will be swollen, painful, and tender to touch. It may not be possible to distinguish a sprain from a

fracture without medical advice.
1. A firm bandage may give relief.
2. The joint should be rested.
3. A medical opinion may be needed if there is much pain or swelling.

Suffocation and strangulation

1. Immediately remove whatever is causing the obstruction or strangulation.
2. If breathing is difficult, or has stopped, begin mouth-to-mouth respiration (see page 175).
3. Seek medical advice without delay.

Sunburn

Children and babies burn very easily. Avoid prolonged exposure to direct sunlight, especially on the coast, where sea breezes give an illusion of coolness. Always remember it takes six to twelve hours for sunburn to develop. Babies benefit from sunhats, and in very hot sun, a screening cream will help.

Once burning has occurred prevent further exposure until recovery. Calamine lotion will offer some relief, and extra fluids should be given to compensate for the increased loss of moisture from the skin.

Sunstroke

Sunstroke is a form of heatstroke. In addition to the general features of heatstroke, there is the problem of sunburn to deal with. In these circumstances, the sunburn may be severe and extensive, with blistering and a loss of fluid and plasma into the blisters.

The warning signs are exhaustion, irritability, headache,

dizziness and cramps. Fluid and salt replacement are vital. A slightly salty drink of no more than half a teaspoon of salt in a pint of water can be offered along with plain water. Keep the child in a cool place. Treat the sunburn. (page 183).

Full sunstroke occurs when the body temperature rises to 104°F/40°C or more. The child is restless, confused or even semiconscious. Urgent cooling is necessary. The child should be stripped naked and wrapped in a cold, wet sheet. Fanning will increase the rate of cooling by evaporation. It may be necessary to repeat the fanning in the cold sheet several times. The child needs urgent transfer to hospital.

Swallowed objects

Small children may inadvertently swallow objects such as buttons, beads and coins they have in their mouths. If the child chokes on an object it may be stuck in the windpipe. See treatment for choking, page 177.

If the object is swallowed there is no immediate anxiety, but medical aid should be sought. Many objects pass through the digestive tract without incident, but some can cause obstruction and require surgical removal.

Toothache

If a child has toothache he will need to see a dentist as a matter or urgency. However at night, or if a dentist is not available, first aid treatment may be necessary.

Toothache is most commonly due to an area of dental decay (caries) involving the nerve in the centre of the tooth. A bud of cotton wool on a stick, dipped into clove oil and then inserted into the

cavity, will temporarily relieve the toothache. Care should be taken not to allow the clove oil to touch anywhere except the cavity. If no oil of cloves is available, or no cavity can be seen, sucking ice may give some relief, as may aspirin or paracetamol.

Traffic accidents

Action on arrival
1. Make sure that someone telephones for emergency services immediately.
2. **Do not** pull the child from the vehicle, unless there is immediate danger of further injury, fire, severe bleeding, or breathing has stopped.
3. Switch the engine off to minimize fire risk.
4. Set up warning triangles or flares, or ask bystanders to direct traffic.
5. Make sure the car cannot roll by placing blocks on either side of the wheels.
6. Check inside the car for any small children or babies who may have fallen out of sight.

Do not move the child if you suspect spinal injuries. Unskilled removal of a child with spinal injuries from a wrecked car may result in permanent and avoidable damage.

If it is absolutely necessary to move the child, do so with particular care. Try to keep the neck and spine still and the head from wobbling. Find somewhere safe, dry and firm for the injured child and do not move again until the ambulance arrives.

On the spot treatment
Bleeding (see page 176).
Fractures (see page 180).
Recovery position (see page 177).
Artificial respiration (see page 173)
Heart massage (see page 174).

Bandaging and the First Aid Box

There should be a variety of different bandages in a First Aid Box. In order not to make mistakes at a time when speed is important it is worth practising trying different types of bandages on friends or members of the family.

Types and specific uses: (see right)
1. Triangular—open and unfolded, as a sling or for securing dressings over areas such as the head, hand and foot. Folded (see broad and narrow bandages below) for securing dressings, immobilizing limbs, securing splints, making a ring pad. **2. Roller**—keeps dressing in position, supports a strain or strain. **3. Sterile unmedicated dressings** — for large wounds. **4. Gauze dressings** — for light covering on burns; or a substitute for sterile unmedicated dressing. **5. Adhesive dressings** — 'plasters', used for covering minor wounds.
Improvised bandages can be made from clean ties, handkerchiefs and scarves.

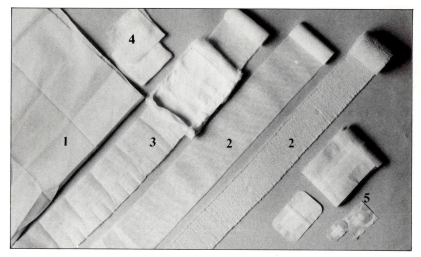

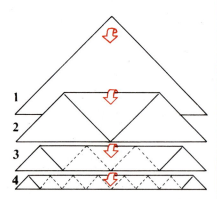

Making broad/narrow bandages
1. To make a broad bandage start with a triangular bandage.
2. Fold the top point of the triangle to the middle of the base.
3. Fold it once more in the same direction.
4. To make a narrow bandage fold the broad bandage in half again in the same direction.

Making a ring bandage

A ring bandage is an open pad which is used to help protect a wound from pressure if, for example, a foreign body is still in wound.

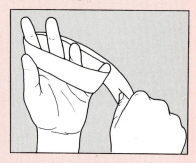

Making a ring pad:
1. Take a narrow bandage and wind it once or twice round your finger to make a loop.

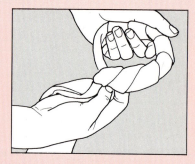

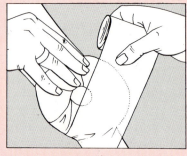

2. Pass the other end of the bandage through the loop, around and through again, until a solid ring has been formed and all the bandage is used up.

3. Place the open pad on the wound and secure it in place with a second bandage, preferably a roller bandage.

184

First aid box

A first aid box should be easily accessible to you, but out of reach of children. High up in a kitchen cabinet is one good place.

Contents

1. Triangular bandages — for making a sling. (A clean, folded nappy might do).

2. Sterilized cotton wool — to clean wounds.

3. Various size packets of sterile gauze dressings.

4. Assorted adhesive plasters — for minor cuts and grazes.

5. Non-adherent absorbent dressings — try to buy the type with a peel-off back. They should be about 4 ins square, and made of gauze.

6. Crepe bandage — used for sprains and muscle strains.

7. Eye pad with bandage — for eye injuries.

8. Scissors.

9. Safety pins.

10. Eye lotion.

11. Surgical tape for sticking down the edges of dressing.

Also

A finger bandage, tweezers, a packet of soluble aspirin, antihistamine cream, a mild disinfectant for cleaning wounds and some antiseptic cream to put on minor cuts.

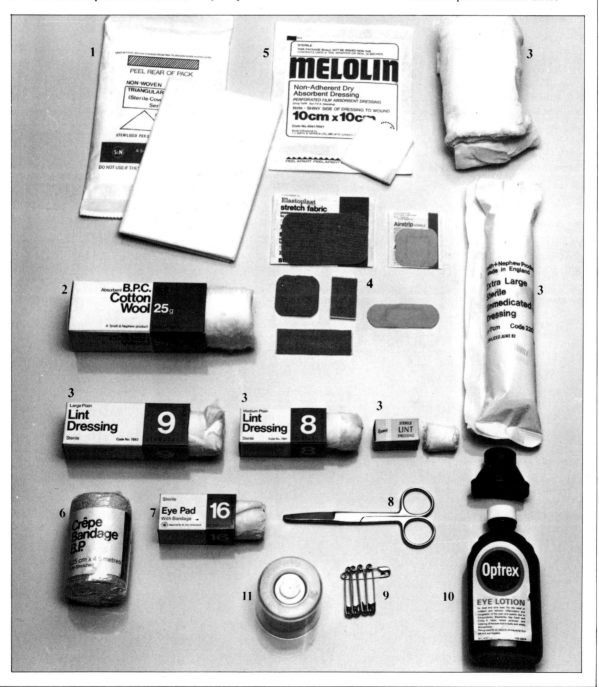

Index

Acknowledgements

Asthma Society and Friends of the Asthma Research
Council, British Diabetic Association, British Epilepsy
Association, Child Accident Prevention Trust, Devilbiss
Health Care UK Ltd, Fisons Ltd (Pharmaceutical
Division), Health Education Council, Holstar Instruments
Ltd, Hospital Equipment and Supplies magazine, Dr M.J.
Goldsmith, Executive Medical Director, The Harrow
Health Care Centre, McCormick Intermarco-Farner Ltd,
National Society for Mentally Handicapped Children and
Adults (MENCAP), Richardson-Vicks Ltd, Royal
National Institute for the Deaf (RNID), St. John
Ambulance Association, Shuco International London Ltd,
Scottish Health Education Group, Vickers Medical

Photography
John Watney Picture Library, London Scientific Fotos,
Mark Richards, Anna Dubbelt, Alistair Campbell,
Edward Kinsey

Special thanks to:
St George's Hospital, Tooting, London

Additional thanks to:
Hilary Arnold, Pat Baldwin, Moira Clinch, Richard
Gough, Pat, Thomas and Nancy Graham, Iain
Hutchinson, Helen Varley, Sarah and Joseph Wyand.